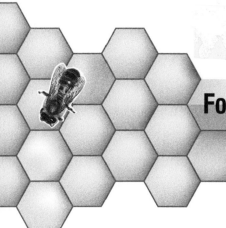

Foundations in Nursing and Health Care

Nursing Numeracy: a new approach

Carol Chapelhow and Sandra Crouch
Series Editor: Lynne Wigens

Nelson Thornes
a Wolters Kluwer business

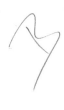
Published in 2007 by:
Nelson Thornes Ltd
Delta Place
27 Bath Road
CHELTENHAM
GL53 7TH
United Kingdom

07 08 09 10 11 / 10 9 8 7 6 5 4 3 2 1

A catalogue record for this book is available from the British Library

ISBN 9780 7487 9681 6

Page make-up by Florence Production Ltd

Printed and bound in Slovenia by Korotan-Ljubljana

Contents

Acknowledgements

We would like to thank the following people who have each in their own way contributed to this book:

Students, too numerous to mention.

Particular thanks go to our husbands and close family, who despite developing a particular 'resigned' look at evenings and weekends, gave us much love, encouragement and support.

Our many friends for their patience and forbearance, as well as for sticking by us.

Professor Vince Ramprogus for all of the support and encouragement he gave us in the early days of our encounters with the numeracy problem.

Our heartfelt thanks to Dr Rosie Crane, a like-minded supporter, and Dr Omar Veledar for his painstaking work to ensure that our number operations/calculations are as correct as they possibly can be.

Thanks also to Mike Sabin, for renewing our enthusiasm and self-belief by confirming that we were on the right track and that developing our approach was, as Schon (1983) so nicely puts it, working in the 'swampy lowlands'.

And, last but not least, thanks to many colleagues who went the extra mile when we were up against deadlines, specifically: Margaret Scott, Sharon Hartley, Malcolm Bell, Michael Kelleher, Carol Grant and Lillian Broatch.

References

Schon, D. (1983) *The reflective practitioner*. London, Temple South.

Introduction

Unfortunately, numeracy is not seen to be sexy. Indeed, it sometimes seems that it is more acceptable to discuss death and cancer in public in our society today than admit to having any difficulties with or interest in numbers. Perhaps that is because, if you do feel that your number skills are not what you think they should be, you feel embarrassed and uncomfortable around the issue of numbers and maths. As a result of such feelings, many people seem to try to avoid engaging with numbers, particularly in public, or at least feel very self-conscious when they have to put their skills up for public view, particularly at work. Yet, while these types of feelings seem to be common, these same people engage in number skills every day but are not fully aware of it. Many people manage a very difficult family budget in a way that the Chancellor of the Exchequer would envy. Some play darts and have no problem instantly counting backwards. Others travel to foreign countries that have different currencies and come back with some real bargains. So they do not have any difficulties with numeracy – or do they?

If you feel embarrassed, humiliated, afraid, ashamed or anxious and panicky when confronted with number, you are not alone; many adults seem to have difficulties with numbers for a variety of reasons. Today, many people rarely use their number skills, mainly because they have little need to. We have machines that do so many calculations, from hand-held calculators to shop tills. As a result, you often get very little opportunity to keep your number skills up to date and, like any other skill, if you do not practise it the skill will fade. The old adage is 'Use it or lose it'.

Some of you will feel that you have some numeracy difficulties, but these may be perceived rather than actual. Many of you will be using this book to satisfy yourself that you do have numeracy skills, while others will turn to it for help in assisting others who are trying to learn nursing numeracy skills.

Apparently no one in nursing has yet explored the factors that inhibit the development of many people's number skills or applied this to how adults learn numeracy best.

This is what this book does, which is why we believe that our approach to nursing numeracy is unique. Our approach also recognises that the difficulties that many people appear to have with numbers can occur across the nursing hierarchy and not just within the student population.

The driver for developing this unique approach is and always has been to enable people to reassure themselves about and/or to develop their number skills. Therefore this book aims to help students as well as qualified health care professionals of all levels. There is no doubt that this is an original way of helping working adults develop their mathematical skills.

If you do have some numeracy difficulties, there are a variety of reasons why you have such problems. We explore some of the common factors such as gender issues and the transferability of skills that appear to be implicated in the development of such difficulties. As the nursing numeracy problem is multi-faceted, our approach takes an innovative stance in helping you to address these factors. As a result, it is not only comprehensive but also different from other books/study guides exploring numeracy that you may have used before. We have written this book for readers who need help to understand the different concepts and who will dip in and dip out. Consequently, while we would like you to read it from cover to cover, each chapter is designed to stand on its own. The book explores the main factors that affect many nurses' perceptions of their numeracy difficulties/anxieties so that you can recognise them and confront the challenge to your competence and/or confidence.

We have written this book to help you develop your numeracy skills. However, during the course of writing, it became very clear that confidence in abilities plays a very important part in how competent you are. So we want to play some part in the way that you develop your numeracy skills and also how you develop your confidence and success. The authorship process has also demonstrated that most people know much more than they realise (Chinn 1998).

As nurses, we are very conscious that we are not mathematicians. However, what we have discovered is that our concerns are the same concerns that mathematicians have. In addressing these concerns our approach recognises that:

- Not everyone uses the same methods
- There may be many alternatives. One may suit you better, so give them a try and find the one that works best for you. All we would ask, in the name of patient safety, is that you check that you have the correct answer, no matter which way you calculate

- Concepts/ideas should be revisited to strengthen your understanding
- Anxiety can be reduced by identifying what you are good at
- Sometimes you have to take risks; you cannot protect yourself from being wrong (Chinn 1998).

This book is designed in such a way that you will have the opportunity to explore and develop your numeracy skills in a non-threatening way, away from the stress of clinical environments. We use patient scenarios to reflect the numbers that many nurses use in their day-to-day work. Using our tools (the Skills checklist and Theory to practice) we set these number skills into the context of nursing work.

This book, and particularly the case studies used in Chapter 2, focuses on research studies presented in the mathematics, ethnomathematics, psychology, education and sociology literature, for example in Evans (2000), Cadinu *et al.* (2003) and Johns, Schmader and Martens (2005).

Remember that both the activities and feedback in this book are private to you. This will enable you to work at your own pace, stimulated by using a variety of relevant, enjoyable and context-based exercises.

You might find it useful to use this book in conjunction with your Professional Portfolio. You will then have a record of your learning and professional development that will count as evidence for the learning activities that you have completed towards the Post Registration Education and Practice (PREP) Continuing Professional Development (CPD) standard, which is part of the requirements for your periodic re-registration with the Nursing and Midwifery Council (NMC 2005).

This book therefore fulfils several purposes:

- It promotes competence and confidence in your existing number skills by exploring examples from everyday life so that you can recognise the number skills you already have
- It provides an easily understood overview of SI units and types of number calculations that nurses use in everyday practice
- It identifies a wide range of contemporary nursing situations in which nurses calculate
- It draws heavily on practice situations so that the applicability of number skills to nursing can be considered
- It identifies which skills you, the user of the book, have problems with, if any, and offers suggestions as to how you may address any deficiencies you might have.

Please note that throughout the book we have tried to reflect current practice. You will notice that some of the calculations do not reflect the SI units involved. This seems to be common practice in clinical areas but the SI units are important, numbers without the units lose their meaning.

References

Cadinu, M., Maass, A., Frigerio, S., Impagliazzo, L. and Latinotti, S. (2003) Stereotype threat: The effect of expectancy on performance. *European Journal of Social Psychology*, **33**, 267–285.

Chinn, S. (1998) *Sum Hope. Breaking the numbers barrier.* Souvenir Press, London.

Evans, J. (2000) *Adult's Mathematical Thinking and Emotions: a Study of Numerate Practices.* Taylor Francis, London.

Johns, M., Schmader, T. and Martens, A. (2005) Knowing is half the battle: teaching stereotype threat as a means of improving women's math performance. *Psychological Science*, **16**(3), 175–179.

Nursing and Midwifery Council (2005) *The PREP Handbook.* NMC, London.

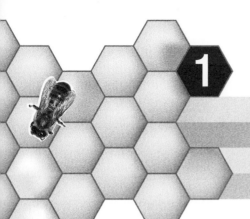

Nursing Numeracy: the changing context of nursing

This chapter explores the relevance of number skills for contemporary nursing practice.

Learning outcomes

By the end of this chapter you should be able to:

- Identify contemporary developments in nursing care
- Identify clinical situations which require number skills
- Discuss factors which influence the successful application of numeracy skills to care

Contemporary developments in care and the introduction of new nursing roles

Nursing has never been clearly and succinctly defined, and in today's National Health Service (NHS) it is becoming ever more fragmented and specialised as nursing is forced to rise to the challenge of the political drivers. As a result, nursing is developing an ever-widening set of roles and functions, which has provoked a debate within the profession as to whether or not nursing is at risk of losing its focus and even its identity (McKenna 2005). Since the rise of the specialist nurse there have been some improvements in the service provided to many patients, particularly those with long-term conditions. For example, nutrition nurse specialists appear to have made an impact in recent years in improving the nutritional status of many hospitalised patients. The development of nursing roles has meant that some skills are being retained by nurses, while new skills are being added to the nurse's repertoire (McKenna 2005; Rolfe 1996). The Chief Nursing Officer (Department of Health 2002a) has identified 10 key roles for nurses that are consistent with developments outlined in *The NHS Plan* (Department of Health 2000) and *Liberating the Talents* (Department of Health 2002b). These roles are:

- To order diagnostic investigations such as pathology tests and X-rays
- To make and receive referrals directly, for example to a therapist or pain consultant
- To admit and discharge patients for specified conditions and within agreed protocols

- To manage patient caseloads, for example for diabetes or rheumatology
- To run clinics, such as for ophthalmology or dermatology
- To prescribe medicines and treatments
- To carry out a wide range of resuscitation procedures including defibrillation
- To perform minor surgery and outpatient procedures
- To triage patients using the latest information technology (IT) to the most appropriate health professional
- To take a lead in the way local health services are organised and in the way that they are run.

Inevitably, these roles will involve identification, interpretation and evaluation, and will therefore necessitate using numerical information.

According to Hewitt-Taylor (2002, p. 52) nursing has become holistic, and involves 'technical and pharmacological interventions or procedures such as endotracheal suctioning or wound dressings'. One of the most challenging developments in nursing has been the advent of nurse prescribing. The supporters of nurses prescribing suggest that nurses are best placed to support service users (Mullally 2002) and improve their concordance/compliance with medicines, which is consistent with current government initiatives (Department of Health 2002c). However, some nurses are concerned about this change in role; they need to be reassured about knowledge and accountability, despite evidence which identifies the potential for improved quality of care. Many nurses are concerned about taking responsibility for prescribing decisions (Hewitt-Taylor 2002). However, what is sometimes overlooked is the role of supplementary prescribing – working within a treatment plan agreed with an independent prescriber. Supplementary prescribing involves providing a wider range of medicines to patients with a broader range of medical conditions.

Not only is the nursing workforce changing and developing, but at the same time technologies of care are also transforming, often in revolutionary ways, impacting on the way that patients are treated and cared for. Although advances in medicine mean that many people now have non-invasive or minimally invasive surgery, many more people now survive major life-threatening events than would have been thought possible even a decade ago (Department of Health 2006). As a result, not only are large numbers of people living with chronic long-term conditions, but patients in hospital are frequently sicker and have shorter hospital stays than ever before (Department of Health 2006).

Allied with this, the environment that many nurses work in is becoming ever more technical. High-technology units such as intensive care units involve an increasing range of calculations for nurses, and nurses are accountable for all of their actions. What complicates the situation is that these calculations are often individual to the patient (Hutton 1998a). It is also important that nurses do not rely completely on the information provided by the equipment they are using, but are able to confirm the readings obtained (Jukes and Gilchrist 2005). Miller (1992) suggests that technology, for example that related to intravenous infusion delivery, means that nurses' numeracy skills have deteriorated because they do not practise them frequently enough. He offers the example of a nurse being able to calculate ml per hour but not drops per minute. The increasing reliance on technology also requires nurses to interpret information which is presented to them in different ways, for example through digital displays.

The NHS Plan (Department of Health 2000) identifies clearly the need to change the service so that it is more responsive to patient needs. In this document the Department of Health spells out the need for a service that is patient led. It also identifies the need for care that is more personalised but which also empowers patients so that they become decision makers. This was followed by the introduction of the White Paper, *The Expert Patient: A New Approach to Chronic Disease Management for the 21st Century* (Department of Health 2001). The key focus of the document is to give patients greater control over their lives and enable them to be partners in their care. In order for these policies to be realised we need to provide information to patients that is not only directly concerned with their condition, but relates also to how to manage that condition; inevitably this will involve some numeracy. Those of us who 'manage' with the numeracy demands in current care delivery will find this a subtle but significant change. Think, for example, about a patient with diabetes mellitus who adjusts their insulin dose in response to their blood sugar levels. Explaining to a patient how to calculate their insulin dose so that they understand and can take over this aspect of their care is challenging even when the patient has good numeracy skills.

Evidence-based care should be the basis of all care delivered within today's health service. Evidence-based practice has developed as a response to care delivery based upon tradition or ritual. There is a wealth of evidence available for us to use, but it is often difficult to discriminate between conflicting evidence or to judge the quality of the evidence. For example, if we aim to 'integrate individual expertise with the best available external clinical evidence from systematic research' (Sackett *et al.* 1996), then we need to be able to interpret research findings, particularly if that research is quantitative. Hek (1994) also identifies numeracy as a requirement in the application of evidence-based practice, one source of which is research. There are other sources of evidence which are qualitative, such as patient views. Evidence-based practice is defined by Chapelhow *et al.* (2005) as 'a way of working, which relies on . . . retrieving and using information from a variety of sources to underpin . . . practice'.

There is evidence to suggest that experienced nurses use previous experience to estimate, for example, the amount of feed required by a baby of a particular weight, rather than consulting theoretical sources (Hutton 1998b). One reason for this is that nurses use subjective assessment and measurement on a regular basis. Nursing does not always lend itself to objectivity – how do you measure care? We can identify examples of objective measurements (e.g. medicine doses, off-duty rotas, mileage) from practice and 'life'. But there are also many instances where subjective measurements are required, such as the use of pain assessment tools. In order to be credible in our professional role we need to use objective measurements, but in some situations, such as urinalysis, a combination of objective and subjective measurements provides a much more comprehensive picture. For example, when carrying out a urinalysis we would measure amount (volume) and we would measure its constituents. Equally important to consider is the colour, smell and presentation, e.g. is it cloudy, does it contain blood? Another example would be when measuring the patient's pulse – rate is important, but we need to qualify this with rhythm and strength.

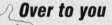

Over to you

Can you identify a range of:

● objective measurements
● subjective measurements

that are frequently used in clinical areas?

Recognising and applying numeracy in nursing care

There seems to be an urban myth that the only numbers used in nursing are those related to the administration of medicines. This appears to be compounded by the nursing literature, as almost all the books and articles that explore mathematical skills in nursing focus on the number skills required to calculate doses of medicine, drip rates for intravenous fluids or, less frequently, the dilution of solutions. There is no doubt that this is a limited approach, which neither effectively equips nurses for the diversity of practice situations in which they will require number skills on a daily basis, nor recognises the breadth of the application of number in nursing. Is it because number is not fully recognised that the focus becomes the only visible numbers in nursing – those associated with medication calculations and intravenous infusions? Our work is distinctive in recognising that there are numbers in nursing other than in medication calculation and intravenous therapy.

Having earlier identified some of the other forms of measurement in nursing, starting with pulse and urinalysis, we can now begin to identify other areas of nursing where measurement and interpretation, and therefore using number systems, are important. Coben and Atere-Roberts (2005) have written a useful book for health care students which goes further than the traditional approaches to numeracy as they also identify fluid balance, infant feeding, staffing and budget calculations, and demographic profiles. We describe some of these and introduce you to a few more below, specifically within the chapters containing the patient scenarios.

However, we do not wish to minimise the importance of calculation related to medicine administration. According to the Department of Health (Department of Health 2004), medication errors cost the NHS between £200 million and £400 million per year. Administration of medicines is a key part of the nurse's role. While there are a number of reasons for mistakes (e.g. problems with prescription errors, workload and staffing issues, and the working environment), it is inevitable that some errors result from nurses' inability to calculate (Trim 2004). This is reiterated by Haigh (2002), who suggests that a major cause of medication errors must be the nurses' poor mathematical abilities. Administration of medicines is undertaken frequently, but according to Kapborg (1994, p. 72) it 'makes both the nurse and patient very vulnerable'. Administration of medicines is a required competency for entry to the professional register (Nursing and Midwifery Council 2004), and therefore we must be both competent and confident in this area.

Nursing numeracy

Having identified that medicine administration errors may occur for a variety of reasons, there have been several research studies in this area which show that nurses have difficulties with mathematical, conceptual (difficulty in setting up the problem) and measurement aspects of the calculation (Trim 2004).

Sometimes the difficulty is with nurses' perceptions of where measurement in nursing occurs. For example, research undertaken by Cartwright (1996) suggests that nurses do not see observation as a form of measurement, and that nurses estimate based upon their experience. Worryingly, Cartwright went on to suggest that nurses also estimated drip rates rather than using a formula. This might be explained by the previous discussion which indicates that nurses frequently use subjective measurements, and if they have concerns about their numeracy they may begin to rely on these, particularly if they have a lot of experience to draw on.

Many authors (Chinn 1998) suggest that 'most people know more maths than they realise'. So why do so many of us doubt our mathematical skills? It might be that we do not recognise that we are using mathematical skills, or that the words used carry a meaning that brings with it anxiety. The terms 'mathematics' and 'mathematical skills' seem to be used quite widely, but within this book we use the terms 'number' and 'number skills' or 'numeracy' to describe the skills of addition, subtraction, division and multiplication that nurses will use in their everyday practice. Our choice of this terminology is supported by the Cockcroft Committee Report (1982, paras. 32–35), which states that numeracy is the 'ability to cope confidently with the mathematical needs of everyday life'. It further suggests that such an ability includes 'a feeling for number' that 'permits sensible estimation and approximation that enables straightforward mental calculation to be accomplished'.

If we consider the statement made by Steve Chinn (1998), it may be that we come to each mathematical situation as if it is new to us, i.e. we do not recognise mathematical principles and so-called tricks that we have used before. In order to build your confidence we want to encourage the *transferability* of numeracy skills. Hence we have used the definition of numeracy offered by Evans (2000), as he seems to support the underlying philosophy that has led us to devise our approach to support the transfer of learning from one situation to another.

Evans (2000, p. 236) defines numeracy as:

> the ability to process, interpret and communicate numerical, quantitative, spatial, statistical, even mathematical information in ways that are appropriate for a variety of contexts, and that will enable a typical member of the culture or subculture to participate in the activities that they value.

Promoting meaningful learning

There are problems recruiting and retaining qualified nurses in British health care. Keighley (2002) goes so far as to suggest that many of these problems are due to society's dislocation from caring. The impact of this is that many health care settings seem to be understaffed and operating with an inappropriate skill mix. Several of these areas seem to rely on a transient workforce. This has potential implications for care if we consider that the society that today's nurses are drawn from is said to be less numerate than it was in the 1800s (Woodhead 2003). Indeed, the Basic Skills Agency (2001) states that 25% of the adult working population cannot read charts or interpret data from lists.

Over to you

If 25% of the adult working population cannot read charts or interpret data from lists, work out what **ratio** of the total adult working population this represents.

Keywords

Ratio
The relationship between two numbers is found by dividing one by another. It is represented by writing the two resulting numbers separated by a colon

Well done if you made the answer 1:4. There are a number of ways that you could have done this calculation:

- In your head or on paper you could have calculated 25/100 = 4. 100 represents the percentage sign in '25%' of the population
- You could have 'seen' immediately in your head that it was 4. Although actually you would have done the calculation in your head very quickly, so quickly that you were not aware of it
- You could have added 25 to itself until you reached 100, counting the number of times you added the 25s together, e.g.

  25 + 25 = 50
  50 + **25** = 75
  75 + **25** = 100

  which makes 4 times.

  REMEMBER – No matter how confident you are in the number you 'see' in your head, nursing calculations must always be checked.

Reflective activity

Spend a few moments thinking about whether 1 in 4 nurses that you know cannot read charts or interpret data from lists.

It is difficult to prove whether this statistic from the Basic Skills Agency can be projected to nursing and therefore really means that 1 in 4 nurses cannot read charts or interpret data from lists. Perhaps all that we can safely say is that there will be some people working as qualified nurses and on pre-registration programmes who will have problems with numeracy, but who they are and how many there are is impossible to say.

Although much of the nursing literature identifies problems such as those described above, appropriate solutions have not been found. A number of studies (Flynn *et al.* 1996; Rice and Bell 2005; Wright 2005) examine the most effective teaching methods by comparing a number of different teaching strategies. Apparently no one in nursing has yet explored the factors that inhibit the development of many people's number skills or applied this to how adults learn numeracy best.

Sabin (2003) seems to be unique in nursing in recognising that in order to address the problem of numeracy within the NHS an alternative approach has to be developed. Like many other employers, the NHS has been trying to find a solution to the problems that are inherent in the adult workforce today and appear to be getting worse year by year (Parliamentary Public Accounts Committee 2006; Shepherd 2006). The ethnomathematicians who are seeking to understand how professionals use numeracy in their working practice seem to be suggesting that an understanding of the context in which the professional operates is fundamental. Indeed, Pozzi, *et al.* (1998) call this process 'mathematisation'.

There are a variety of problems that many people have with numbers and mathematics. The education, psychology, sociology, mathematics and ethnomathematic disciplines all lean towards a growing acceptance that mathematical and numerate thinking has to be observed and understood in context. Among these groups there is also a suggestion that everyday numerical thinking used in different work situations is different in different contexts. Much of the literature on the numeracy skills of working adults, both national and international, was written in the 1980s and 1990s; some of this is seminal work. What it highlights is how workplace mathematics differs from that taught in school, and the little use it makes of formal approaches (Fahrmeier 1984; Masingila 1993; Nunes *et al.* 1993; Saxe 1991; Scribner 1984, 1985, 1986; Pozzi, Ness and Hoyles 1998).

The poor numeracy skills affecting large numbers of people across the adult workforce seem to have started to become apparent in the 1980s. Subsequently, causes have been suggested and a number of strategies have been introduced at various times, none of which have been particularly successful. The primary concern is numeracy in the adult working population; this means doctors, accountants and engineers as well as nurses, porters and administrators. Although the teaching of mathematics in schools is thought to have changed somewhat over the last 10 years or more, there is little evidence that this has had any major impact on the young adults joining the workforce. The evidence to date seems to suggest that the strategies that have been implemented have only been implemented in some schools, and have been far from successful (Qualifications and Curriculum Authority 2005). Indeed, the National Research and Development Centre research cited in the Qualifications and Curriculum Authority Mathematics: 2004/5 Annual Report (2005, p. 18) states that 'there is an emphasis in the curriculum on memorising mathematical information rather than on understanding mathematical concepts and using mathematical reasoning'. Interestingly, *The Times Higher Education Supplement* (10 February 2006) leaked the results of a survey carried out by researchers at Oxford University and UCAS of the Oxbridge, Russell Group and post-1992 institutions that highlight the lack of basic numeracy (and literacy) skills in A level students, which they say is much worse than it was 10 years ago. They are cited as saying this was because 'Learners who may have achieved academic success by such means at A level . . . are increasingly coming into higher education expecting to be told the answers.' They suggest that the main reason for this is that learning and teaching are assessment driven and generally students are not encouraged to be independent learners.

As nurses are representative of today's adult working population, difficulties with number skills must be manifest in all levels of the qualified nursing workforce. Consequently there must be very senior nurses as well as very recently qualified staff nurses who are very concerned not only about their number skills, but also that other people may notice that their number skills are not quite up to scratch. If this is the case it would go some way to explaining why there are very few research studies exploring mathematical ability in qualified nurses. It becomes even more important to ensure that all people, including those in more senior positions, who do have concerns about their mathematical ability, are given support to overcome any weaknesses in their number skills.

Although many people have anxieties about their number skills, this does not mean that they are not numerate. People appear to have such anxieties for a variety of reasons. Firstly, numeracy is a skill and, as with any other skill, you become less proficient if you do not practise it. Just like riding a bike, if you do not keep riding, you become less proficient, so that when you get on the bike again it takes a little practice in order to regain your original skill level. So, if you are unexpectedly presented with some unusual calculations, you may feel anxious about whether you will be able to do them correctly.

Although medicine calculations are one of the numeracy skills required by nurses, there are many more situations where nurses use number skills. The rationale for including more than medicine calculations here is that nurses routinely use number skills in many aspects of their daily work. Nurses, like most working adults, need to have a set of number skills that they can use in any work situation. They need to be able to use number in whichever clinical situation they find themselves, whether that is fluid balance, budgeting, audit, analysing statistics or calculating medicine dosage using body weight. For a number of years it has been assumed that people are able to transfer the skills they learned from school mathematics lessons to their work environment. However, it has been suggested (Bransford *et al.* 1989; Sierpinska 1994) that the transfer of learning is not automatic and that many people are not able to easily transfer skills from one area to another. This may be because 'the same set of circumstances may not seem [that] similar to other people' (Bransford *et al.* 1989, p. 479).

Thus for many people the traditional way of teaching mathematics in school has not equipped them with the number skills that they need in their workplace, nor has it given them the skills to enable them to transfer their learning from school to work. The people who admit that they have difficulty with number skills therefore need to be given the opportunity to develop their numeracy skills in a different way. Chapter 2 highlights some of the factors that might have influenced the way that some people view their numeracy skills, while the patient scenarios in Chapters 7–10 will show how numeracy skills can be transferred from one situation to another.

Conclusions

In this chapter we have explored the changes to nursing roles and care delivery that have highlighted the need for accurate measurement and interpretation of numbers. We have shown that numeracy is inherent in the activities a nurse undertakes on a daily basis and identified some examples of this. However, we have also identified that there are growing concerns about the numeracy skills of the general population. We suggest that current approaches to numeracy are not helpful to nurses as they do not contextualise the problems effectively or provide strategies to facilitate the transfer of skills from one clinical context to another.

RRRRRRapid recap

Check your progress so far by working through each of the following points:

1. Identify some areas in care delivery where we need to use objective measurements
2. Suggest two reasons why nurses might be concerned about their numeracy skills
3. Identify some current initiatives in nursing which will require a greater awareness of numeracy
4. Identify the underpinning philosophy for this new approach to numeracy

If you have difficulty with more than one of the questions, read through the section again to refresh your understanding before moving on.

References

Bransford, J.D., Franks, J.J., Vye, N.J. and Sherwood, R.D. (1989) New approaches to instruction: because wisdom can't be told. In: *Similarity and Analogical Reasoning* (eds. Vosniadou, S. and Ortony, A.). Cambridge University Press, Cambridge and New York.

Cartwright, M. (1996) Numeracy needs of the beginning Registered Nurse. *Nurse Education Today*, **16**, 137–143.

Chapelhow, C., Crouch, S., Fisher, M. and Walsh, A. (2005) *Uncovering Skills for Practice*. Nelson Thornes, Cheltenham.

Chinn, S. (1998) *Sum Hope. Breaking the numbers barrier.* Souvenir Press, London.

Coben, D. and Atere-Roberts, E. (2005) *Calculations for Nursing and Healthcare*, 2nd edn. Palgrave Macmillan, Basingstoke.

Department of Education and Science (1981) *Mathematics Counts: report of the Committee of Inquiry into the teaching of mathematics in schools under the chairmanship of Dr. W.H. Cockcroft*. Department of Education and Science.

Department of Health (2000) *The NHS Plan*. Department of Health, London.

Department of Health (2001) *The Expert Patient: a New Approach to Chronic Disease Management for the 21st Century*. Department of Health.

Department of Health (2002a) *Developing Key Roles for Nurses and Midwives: A Guide for Managers*. Department of Health, London.

Department of Health (2002b) *Liberating the Talents: Helping Primary Care Trusts and Nurses to Deliver the NHS Plan*. Department of Health, London.

Department of Health (2002c) *Pharmacists will prescribe for the first time. Nurses will prescribe for chronic illness*. Press release.

Department of Health (2004) *Building a Safer NHS for Patients: Improving Medication Safety*. Department of Health, London.

Department of Health (2006) *Our choice, Our health, Our say: a new direction for community services.* www.dh.gov.uk.

Evans, J. (2000) *Adult's Mathematical Thinking and Emotions: a Study of Numerate Practices.* Taylor Francis, London.

Fahrmeier, E. (1984) Taking inventory: counting as problem solving. *Quarterly Newsletter of the Laboratory of Comparative Human Cognition,* **6**, 6–10.

Flynn, E.R., Wolf, Z.R., McGoldrick, T.B., Seeger Jablonski, R.A., Dean, L.M and McKee, E.P. (1996) Effect of three teaching methods on nursing staff's knowledge of medication risk reduction strategies. *Journal of Nursing Staff Development,* **12**(1), 19–26.

Haigh, S. (2002) How to calculate drug dosage accurately: advice for nurses. *Professional Nurse,* **18**, 54–56.

Harper, N. and Rolfe, S. (1995) Ability of hospital doctors to calculate drug dosages. *British Medical Journal,* **310**, 1173–1174.

Hek, G. (1994) Adding up the cost of teaching mathematics. *Nursing Standard,* **8**(22), 25–29.

Hewitt-Taylor, J. (2002) Evidence-based practice. *Nursing Standard,* **17**, 47–52.

House of Commons Comittee of Public Acounts (2006) *Skills for Life: improving adults' literacy and numeracy.* (21st report of session 05–06). The Stationery Office, London. www.publications.parliament.uk/pa/cm200506/cmselect/cmpubacc/792/792.pdf

Hutton, B.M. (1998a) Nursing mathematics: the importance of application. *Nursing Standard,* **13**(11), 35–38.

Hutton, B.M. (1998b) Numeracy skills for intravenous calculations. *Nursing Standard,* **12**(43), 49–53.

Jarvis, P. (1995) *Adult and Continuing Education*, 2nd edn. Routledge, London.

Jukes, L. and Gilchrist, M. (2005) Concerns about numeracy skills of student nurses. *Nurse Education in Practice,* **6**(4), 192–198.

Kapborg, I.D. (1995) An evaluation of Swedish nurse students' calculation ability in relation to their earlier educational background. *Nurse Education Today* **15**, 69–74.

Keighley, T. (2002) As a result of our social dislocation (editorial). *Nursing Management,* **9**(3), 3.

Masingila, J.O. and Moellwald, F.E. (1993) Using Polya to foster a classroom environment for real world problem solving. *School Science and Mathematics,* **5** (807), 245.

Miller, J. (1992) Can nurses do their sums? *Nursing Times,* **88**(32), 58–59.

McIntosh, S. and Vignoles, A. (2001) Measuring and assessing the impact of basic skills on labour market outcomes. *Oxford Economic Papers – A New Series,* **53**(3), 453–481.

McKenna, H. (2005) Commentary: dynamic effects of nursing roles with changing healthcare services. *Journal of Research in Nursing* **10**(1), 99–106.

Mullally, S. (2002) Nurses of all levels can improve patients' experience of health care. *British Journal of Nursing* **11**(7), 424.

Nunes, T., Schliemann, A.D. and Carraher, D.W. (1993) *Street Mathematics and School Mathematics.* Cambridge University Press, Cambridge.

Nursing and Midwifery Council (2004) *Guidelines for the Administration of Medicines.* NMC, London.

Parrish, D. (1998) One day, my son, all these key skills will be yours. *New Statesman*, 13 Nov, **127**(4411), XXI.

Pirie, S. (1987) *Nurses and Mathematics: Deficiencies in Basic Mathematical Skills among Nurses*. Royal College of Nursing, London.

Pozzi, S., Ness, R. and Hoyles, C. (1998) Tools in Practice: mathematics in use. *Educational Studies in Mathematics*, **36**, 105–122.

Qualifications and Curriculum Authority (2005) Mathematics: 2004/5 annual report on curriculum and assessment. QCA/05/2171. www.qca.org.uk/downloads/qca-05-2171-ma-report.pdf.

Rice, J.N. and Bell, M.L. (2005) Using multi-dimensional analysis to improve drug dosage calculation ability. *Journal of Nursing Education*, **44**(7), 315–318

Rolfe, G. (1996) *Closing the Theory-Practice Gap: A New Paradigm for Nursing*. Butterworth-Heinemann, Oxford.

Sabin, M. (2003) *Competence in practice-based calculation: issues for nursing education, a critical review of the literature*. LTSN, Centre for Health Sciences, Higher Education Academy. www.health.academy.ac.uk/publications/occasionalpaper/occasionalpaper03.pdf

Sackett, D. *et al.* (1996) Evidence based medicine: what it is and what it isn't. *British Medical Journal*. **312**(7023), 71–72.

Saxe, G.B. (1991) *Culture and Cognitive Development: Studies in Mathematical Understanding*. Lawrence Erlbaum Associates, Hillsdale.

Scholes, J. (2003) Editorial. *Nursing in Critical Care* **8**(3), 93–95.

Scribner, S. (1984) Studying working intelligence. In: *Everyday cognition: its development in social context* (eds Rogoff, B. and Lave, J). Harvard University Press, Cambridge.

Scribner, S. (1985) Knowledge at work. *Anthropology and Education Quarterly*, **16**, 199–206.

Scribner, S. (1986) Thinking in action: some characteristics of practical thought. In: *Practical intelligence: nature and origins of competence in the everyday world* (eds Sternberg, R.J. and Wagner, R.K.). Harvard University Press, Cambridge.

Shepherd, J. (2006) Tutors in despair at illiterate freshers. *The Times Higher Education Supplement*, 10 February. www.thes.co.uk.

Sierpinska, A. (1994) *Understanding in Mathematics*. Falmer Press, London.

Tariq, V.N.(2002) A decline in numeracy skills among bioscience undergraduates. *Journal of Biological Education*, **36**(2), 76–83.

Tobias, S. (1978) *Overcoming Math Anxiety*. Norton, New York.

Trim, J. (2004) Clinical skills: a practical guide to working out drug calculations. *British Journal of Nursing*, **13**(10), 602–607.

Walkerdine, V. (1998) *Counting Girls Out: Girls and Mathematics*. Falmer Press, London.

Weeks, K. (2000) Written drug dosage errors made by students: the threat to clinical effectiveness. *Clinical Effectiveness in Nursing*, **4**(4), 20–29.

Woodhead, C. (2002) *The Standards of Today*. Adam Smith Institute, London.

Wright, K. (2005) An exploration into the most effective way to teach drug calculation skills to nursing students. *Nurse Education Today*, **25**, 430–436.

2

It must be me! Recognising and dealing with some of the common factors that can affect numeracy performance

Learning outcomes

By the end of this chapter you should be able to:

- Identify which factors, if any, influence your approach to numeracy
- Select suitable strategies to help you begin to develop your numeracy skills
- Recognise some of the influences that may affect your perceptions of your numerical ability

Introduction

It is not unusual to feel anxious or concerned about using numeracy skills in your day-to-day work, especially if you do not use your number skills very often. However, as adults we can all be confident that we possess some number skills.

Over to you

When you decided to buy this book no doubt you first worked out whether you could afford to buy it. Did you:

- Check whether it was cheaper to buy at a bookshop or online?
- Add in the cost of postage when comparing the online price with the bookshop price?
- Check your finances to see whether you could afford it?

If you answered 'yes' to all of the questions in *Over to you*, then you already use the skills of addition and subtraction and are able to compare and analyse numbers. These are very useful skills in budgeting. However, you may be aware of the current debate in the media about the general decline in the numeracy skills of school leavers (Shepherd 2006). This relates to all professional and non-professional groups, but there is also considerable literature relating this to health care professionals. This does not necessarily imply that nurses cannot carry out number calculations successfully. What it probably does mean is that strategies you have been using, or indeed have been taught, are not effective, or cannot be transferred into new environments, e.g. from school to work. Unfortunately this may make you anxious, even though in other situations you have been able to carry out quite complex calculations. Therefore, it is important that you recognise what strengths you have and build upon them. Confidence, according to the theorists, can have a substantial impact on your ability to calculate in a particular situation.

If you feel uneasy when you have to carry out a calculation, or if you feel worried about how well you will cope when you have to calculate something, then you know how this feels. If you have anxieties/concerns about your numeracy skills, then this chapter will help you to recognise the factors that might have led to you being anxious and it will help you to deal with the fears that are blocking your skills. If you are not sure whether you have anxieties/concerns about your mathematical/numeracy skills, you can find out by using the test in the Reflective activity box. Maths anxiety is not the only factor that appears to affect people's *perceptions* of their numerical abilities. The purpose of this chapter, therefore, is to explore not only the factors that may have influenced your perceptions of your numeracy skills, but also those factors that may have influenced how numerate you are.

Reflective activity

How anxious are you about your numeracy skills?

- Do you avoid becoming involved in calculations?
- Do you feel uneasy about doing any kind of calculation?
- Are you frightened of asking questions about calculations?
- Are you worried that you may be asked to explain how you have calculated something?
- Do you avoid having to explain calculations to patients?
- Do you feel that you understand when calculations are explained to you, but when you try to apply this it is as though you never heard the explanation?
- Do you feel that you do not know how to develop your numeracy skills?
- Do you feel as though you are swimming through treacle when you are faced with learning to calculate?

How did you score? If you have answered 'yes' to all eight of the questions then you really are anxious about your skills. This chapter of the book is definitely for you. If you have answered 'yes' to some of these questions, then you will find the following chapter helpful.

Remember, many people feel anxious about their numeracy skills. So it is important at this point to explore some of the issues that might have influenced not only how skilled you are in number, but also how you feel about your abilities in this field. There are some very valid reasons for doing this. Although there is no doubt that competence in numeracy is extremely important, it is also evident that your mind-set is just as important. Indeed, magnetic resonance imaging (MRI) demonstrates this quite clearly. Your emotions can and do influence how you think (Taylor 2001) – negative emotions can interfere with your performance (Ashcraft and Kirk 2001; Ashcraft 2002; Evans 2000; Hopko *et al.* 2003; Trbovich and LeFevre 2003). Of the books currently on the UK market that aim to help nurses develop their numeracy skills, most focus largely on number skills. But here we will explore your numerical competence; your attitudes, emotions and resulting self-confidence in relation to numeracy; as well as how professionals apply numeracy to their field of practice.

There is much research evidence to suggest that there are several factors that have an impact on people's numeracy skills. These include: gender, transferability of skills, teachers' attitudes, the fact that school mathematics is not the same as the mathematics used in the workplace, maths anxiety, social class and race. Not all of these factors are explored below, but we will introduce those that appear to have the greatest impact on the majority of nurses.

The image of mathematics

One factor that appears to have had a major impact on how well adults perform numeracy skills is that of gender. There is a large body of research that has concluded that girls and women perform less well than boys and men in mathematics and the pure sciences. It has been suggested that this is why there are relatively few women working in areas that utilise mathematics and science. So strong have been the arguments that such ideas are almost one of today's urban myths. A good example of this occurred in January 2005 when the then president of Harvard University (one of the USA's leading universities) is reported to have said in a speech that 'boys outperformed girls on high school science and maths scores because of genetic differences' (Goldenberg 2005).

Needless to say, arguments such as those expressed by the Harvard University president are disputed vigorously, and not only by the female academic members of staff at Harvard University. It is suggested (Walkerdine 1998; Evans 2000; Baron-Cohen 2004; Kendrick 2005) that the difference in the performance of the sexes is not because there are major differences in the abilities of girls and boys/women and men. Yes, some are more able than others, but this applies equally to both boys and girls. It seems that inherent in producing the difference in mathematical performance between the sexes is the socialisation process of children in school, from nursery school to sixth form (Walkerdine 1998; Evans 2000; Women and Work Commission 2006). Firstly, there are a number of issues related to gender that seem to have had an effect on girls in particular. These seem to revolve around the conflict between femininity and mathematics and science. While there is no doubt that society and the way that we are socialised has changed markedly over the last 20–30 years, this does not seem to have affected our values and beliefs equally. Society still seems to hold dear the more traditional models of femininity and masculinity. Indeed, a report recently published by the Women and Work Commission (February, 2006) draws attention to studies that demonstrate primary-school children clearly verbalising gender stereotypes, showing that such beliefs are formed very early in one's life. Women and girls in Western societies seem to be constantly drip fed this viewpoint and as a result many come to believe that this is indeed so. This seems to be particularly so if you have the slightest doubt about your numerical abilities (Davies *et al.* 2002; Foels and Pappas 2004; Schmader *et al.* 2004; Johns *et al.* 2005).

This chapter considers gender issues that may influence both male and female health care professionals, although it may seem initially to be targeted mainly at women. This is for two reasons:

- Nursing is still a female-dominated profession (Davies 1998) with 89·25% women on the professional register and only 10·75% men (Nursing and Midwifery Council 2005)

- There is currently minimal research literature on the difficulties that men and boys face; perhaps this is because they are not perceived to have many problems with numeracy. However, the problems that are known will be highlighted.

Gender stereotyping

The following activities may reveal some interesting attitudes. Indeed, you may not be aware that you have these attitudes until you carry out the activities.

> ### Over to you
>
> Write down the first four words that come into your head when you think of the word 'feminine'.

The following words are often used to describe 'feminine': soft, nice, warm, appealing, emotional, cute, modest, pure, refined, sensitive, gentle, girly, tender, delicate, dependent, weak and submissive, victim, passive.

> ### Over to you
>
> Name two activities that often seem to be stereotypically linked to being female.

In contrast to men, girls and women are often said to enjoy, among other things, 'shop til' they drop', dressing up, helping children and 'making over' rooms. In addition, girls and women are often viewed as being emotional, irrational and impractical. Indeed, the word 'hysteria' is rooted in the feminine, as it comes from the Greek word *husterikor*, meaning 'of the womb' (*Concise Oxford Dictionary* 2005).

> ### Over to you
>
> Write down the first words that you think of when you think about mathematics and science.

Mathematics and science are frequently represented by adjectives such as objective, rational, hard, cold, calculating, unbiased, dispassionate and detached – words that are also used to describe being male or masculine. These adjectives seem to be the opposite of those used to describe women and femininity.

It therefore seems that in everyday language people are being constantly bombarded with subtle messages that suggest that femininity and being female are conflicting attributes not only to those of men and masculinity, but also to those related to mathematics and the sciences. However, as noted above, the features of mathematics and science seem to be reflected in the virtues of being male and masculine.

It is no wonder that Walkerdine (1998) concluded that girls grow up having to resolve the hidden conflict between performing well in mathematics and science and being feminine. As a result many feel, subconsciously, that mathematics and science are not for them. Many writers and researchers suggest that our society endorses this socialisation of girls and women. Indeed, Walkerdine and Sichtermann (1986), among others, argue that the prevailing way of looking at our society is from a masculine perspective. This perspective on life is so subtle and so entrenched as to be almost invisible, so much so that many people do not realise that they are taking such a biased view. Our individual attitudes, values and beliefs are strongly influenced by those of our society. While such stereotypes are thought to be useful to people when faced with new situations and changing environments, they can be misused without our being aware of it as they can fuel our prejudices (Bar-Tal and Guinote 2002). One aspect of stereotyping which seems to be particularly important in relation to numeracy skills is that of **stereotype threat**.

Stereotype threat seems to be an important concept to consider in relation to numeracy skills in women. A number of research studies (including Cadinu *et al.* 2003; Schmader *et al.* 2003; Foels and Pappas 2004; Keonig and Eagly 2005; McIntyre *et al.* 2005) suggest that stereotype threat appears to reduce the capacity of working memory. The consequence of this is that there is less working memory available to carry out numerical calculations (Ashcraft *et al.* 1998; Hopko *et al.* 2003; Sohn and Doane 2003).

For men in the health professions, and nursing in particular, the influences seem to have been slightly different. These pressures will be explored in relation to what is seen to be an essential attribute of the health care professions – caring.

○━▶ *Keywords*

Stereotype threat
The social and psychological feelings that affect members of a group. These feelings make individual group members underperform relative to their ability

---

> ## *Over to you*
>
> Write down the first four words that come into your head when you think of the word 'masculine'.

When boys and men are referred to as masculine this often infers that they are: stoical, resilient, hardy, strong, robust, tough, resourceful, independent, vigorous, spatially aware, logical, aggressive, single-minded, dominant and active.

> ## Over to you
>
> Name two activities that seem to be stereotypically linked to being masculine.

Many activities still seem to be perceived as mostly male activities. Several of these relate to particular sports such as fishing, rugby, football and motor racing. Motorcycling is also still perceived as a masculine activity, despite its increasing popularity with women.

It has been suggested that male stereotypical attributes can be classified into aspects of power, e.g. independence and leadership, while those of women can be categorised in the characteristics of emotionality, e.g. dependence and nurturing (Allison *et al.* 2004; Davies 1998). Although in Western society these types of male attributes appear to give men greater advantage when pursuing career choices, they are not the attributes that the general public associate with nurses. Caring is seen as fundamental not only to nursing, but also to other health care professions. However, caring has often been described as both an inborn ability as well as a feminine value (Reverby 1987; Warelow 1996), and White (2002) reminds us that the qualities credited to nursing and nurses are also those that are seen to be central to those of mothering and mothers. Such characteristics include the ideals of nurturing, altruism and service. These features appear to be in sharp contrast to those identified above as male and masculine. Although the evidence is sparse (Clarke and O'Neill 2001; Whittock and Leonard 2003; Allison *et al.* 2004), it suggests that Western society seems to hold some very negative stereotypical views about men in nursing.

Male/female brain

Such stereotypical views of men and women are apparently not new. Davies *et al.* (2002) cites a quotation from Socrates, the ancient Greek philosopher (in Bloom 1968), in which Socrates says that men do everything better than women other than feminine activities such as cooking and weaving. As recently as 2004, Foels and Pappas asserted that 'gender socialisation is an arbitrary distinction that socialises men towards dominance and women towards nurturance' (p. 756). Therefore, it is somewhat disconcerting that, as Davies *et al.* (2002) point out, male/female stereotyping seems to have survived unchanged for 2,500 years. This stereotyping seems to stem from the argument that men and women are different because their brains differ. Huge numbers of research studies have been carried out in this area over the years. A considerable number of books and articles have also been published explaining the ideas and thoughts of many people, some experts in their fields and others not, with some propounding very strange ideas. Below is a very concise précis of our understanding of the current reliable and valid scientific findings.

What seems to be key in these research studies is that there are clear differences in functioning between the left and right hemispheres of the human brain. From this evidence it is beginning to appear that there are two types of brain: one type of brain where the right hemisphere is dominant and one kind where the left hemisphere is dominant. As the brain in which the left hemisphere is dominant seems to have more of the characteristics that Western society deems to be female, it is no surprise to find that it has been named the 'female' brain. The opposite holds true for the brain in which the right hemisphere is dominant, which is consequently named the 'male' brain (Baron-Cohen 2004; Kendrick 2005).

While most of these experts agree that it is difficult to separate 'nature' from 'nurture', the studies make it clear that 'any variation in any particular skill or trait within a sex is normally greater than between them' (Baron-Cohen 2004; Kendrick 2005). Or as we said above, some people are more able than others, but this applies equally to boys and girls. So, as with other skills, some men are equally as competent as some women, and some men are equally as incompetent as some women. The other key message is that not all males have male-type brains and not all females have female-type brains. As Kendrick (2005) says: 'variations at brain level are much more complex than that of deciding sex by what you like or which types of sexual organs that you have'. However, there is a school of thought that proposes that the left brain is more analytical than the right brain, while the right brain is considered to use a more holistic methods of thinking about and organising information. Consequently, it would seem that if you have more of a male brain than a female brain your learning style will reflect this, and vice versa.

Over to you

If you would like to find out whether you have a left or right brain there is a test you can take. It is available at http://web.tickle.com/tests/brain/index_main.jsp.

Whether having a left or right brain has any impact on your learning style is hotly debated by theorists. The left/right brain test will identify which type of brain you have, while Chapter 3 might help you to clarify your learning style.

So while it appears that some people have better mathematical skills than others, the reasons for this are not as clear cut as gender stereotyping would have us believe. However, it is becoming clear that gender stereotyping can influence a person's performance in relation to their mathematical abilities. Women, it would seem, feel this more than men.

Feelings, attitudes and expectations

While medicine in the UK has traditionally followed a philosophy that recognises the physical aspects of the body as separate from the mind, many people believe that there is a strong mind–body relationship. Interestingly there seems to be an increasing body of evidence from a recently formed science to support this view. This relatively new science studies the links between three systems: the mind, the immune system and the neurological system. Hence the science is known as 'psychoneuroimmunology'. The scientists working in this field seem to be discovering the emotional molecules that influence not only the way our minds work, but also the immune system and the nervous system (Pert 1999).

There has been much research, argument and debate by psychologists, psychoanalysts, philosophers and doctors over the centuries, but it seems that we are still a long way from being able to define what 'the mind' is or where a thought comes from. Despite this we are able to learn and memorise new things. We use our conscious mind while we are learning, and then store what has been learned in our unconscious mind. However, we are not aware of all that has been stored in our unconscious mind. The unconscious mind can be a repository of unwanted feelings that you are neither aware of nor know where they came from.

Indeed, Taylor (2001, p. 218) suggests that:

'recent research not only provides support that emotions can affect the processes of reason, but more importantly, emotions have been found to be indispensable for rationality to occur. Furthermore, brain research brings to light new insights about a form of long-term memory that has long been overlooked, that of implicit memory, which receives, stores, and recovers outside the conscious awareness of the individual. From implicit memory emerges habits, attitudes and preferences inaccessible to conscious recollection but these are nonetheless shaped by former events, influence our present behaviour, and are an essential part of who we are.'

One such type of feeling inherent in some people's implicit memory seems to be that of mathematics anxiety; this also seems to feature prominently in research related to numeracy difficulty in women. There are very few studies exploring numeracy difficulties in men, perhaps because men are not perceived by our society to have such problems (Aronson *et al.* 1999; Smith and White 2002). Interestingly the one published study to explore whether stereotyping in men affected their mathematical performance demonstrated very clearly that reinforcing negative stereotypes about white men considerably reduced their ability to perform in a maths test (Aronson *et al.* 1999). What is clearly and repeatedly demonstrated in all of the studies exploring maths anxiety in women is that women who are anxious about their numerical skills perform less well in maths tests (Davies *et al.* 2002; Ford *et al.* 2004; Johns *et al.* 2005; McIntyre *et al.* 2005). Ford *et al.* (2004, p. 643) propose that this is because 'women have the added burden of contending with the possibility that their performance might confirm the stereotype of female inferiority and that they might be judged according to that stereotype'.

In the following section we explore the impact that maths anxiety can have, and why some people develop it. If you have mathematics anxiety, it is not always clear why you have it, but it is thought to be related to gender stereotyping (Aronson *et al.* 1999; Ford *et al.* 2004; Schmader *et al.* 2004; Johns *et al.* 2005; McIntyre *et al.* 2005). If you are affected by maths anxiety, later in this chapter you will find some useful strategies that you can use to help you overcome these feelings.

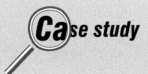

Case study

Angela: Commonly used coping strategies

Outwardly Angela is a competent, confident and outgoing 34-year-old graphic artist, yet she feels very unsure of her mathematical skills. She lives with her husband, Jamie and their son, David, aged 6. At school, when she was considering her career options, she was relieved that she had some artistic flair as it meant that she could pursue an artistic career rather than a science-based one. Neither her husband, a financial adviser, nor her father, an accountant, let her pay for anything. Indeed, Angela never deals with anything around the home that needs any kind of calculation or application of science.

She never checks bills/invoices, bank statements or credit card statements and she never makes a rough estimate of how much the bill will be in the supermarket when she does her weekly shop. When out for a meal with friends she always goes to the toilet when the bill arrives. Then, on her return to the table, she asks what she owes and pays that without checking the bill. While shopping she may compare prices, but only when it is obvious that she is comparing like with like. When she thinks she might have to do some kind of calculation in front of people she feels very anxious and sometimes comes out in a cold sweat.

During Angela's adult life she has unconsciously devised a number of strategies to help her deal with her belief that she cannot do sums.

Over to you

What strategies does Angela use in her day-to-day life when she is faced with having to use numeracy skills?

Keywords

Defence mechanism

A term employed in psychology to describe a strategy used unconsciously by an individual to prevent feelings of anxiety when they perceive themselves to be under threat

Angela's case study illustrates the psychological concepts of both avoidance and denial (Niven 2000). It is thought that many people use these **defence mechanisms** to help them to cope with negative feelings. Such strategies can be seen as negative coping strategies as they will not help Angela address her perceived problem, nor will they help her to be more numerate. Indeed, Angela may only think that she has numeracy problems; she may well be more numerate than she thinks. As was identified earlier in this chapter, stereotype threat such as Angela perceives will reduce her available working memory. Because much of her working memory will be tied up with her anxieties and coping strategies, this leaves little working memory to solve problems. Consequently, when she does engage with a numeracy problem, her error rate will be quite high. This will continually reinforce her belief not only that she cannot do sums, but also the stereotype that women are not mathematically inclined.

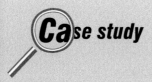

Case study

Kelly: Mathematics anxiety and the influence on lifestyle

Kelly lives with Drew, her partner of 13 years, and their two children. Drew is a self-employed kitchen fitter and Kelly has two part-time jobs. She works for Drew doing administration and accounts, and she works for a local travel agent. Kelly and Drew have a mortgage, an old car that they are buying with a bank loan, and they send both children to a private school. They rarely have any money for anything other than essentials. However, they both pride themselves on being able to manage their money well.

They sometimes go shopping together for groceries and they each make a great show of comparing the prices of similar items in the supermarket. They always buy the item that has the cheaper price tag.

> **Over to you**
>
> Is buying an item based on the cheapest price the best way to obtain value for money?
>
> Why would anyone buy something that was actually more expensive, particularly if money was tight?

Keywords

Avoidance

A psychological term used to explain behaviour that prevents someone doing something. Rather than engage with a particular behaviour, they will always try and escape it

If you are worried about money, your primary concern when shopping is what it will cost at the till when you come to pay. You know that you have finite resources and consequently know how much or how little you can afford to pay. As a result many people buy items that are not best value for money and may be more expensive (Evans 2000). Theorists suggest that if you are constantly anxious about money and are presented with calculations related to finance, you will use the same psychological strategy of avoidance each time you are faced with similar financial calculations, just as Drew and Kelly do when shopping. In other words, even though you may well do the calculations and know that brand X is better value for money than any of the other brands, when you know that you only have a limited amount of money to spend, your emotions can and do prevail over your reason.

This then becomes buried in your unconscious mind, and rather than produce lots of negative emotions and feelings when presented with similar situations, you will use the defence mechanism of avoidance just as Drew and Kelly do because it causes less emotional pain/distress. Indeed, Evans's (2000) study highlights the impossibility of separating our emotions from what we know. Many people feel personal financial pressures, like Kelly and Drew do, and as a result theorists suggest that the emotional factors make them feel that they cannot do sums – consequently they seem to use **avoidance** in all numerical situations.

Comparing the price per quantity of an item ensures that you get best value for money. However, while on a personal level this may be acceptable behaviour, if you are responsible for spending public money wisely, this behaviour may not always be so acceptable. Indeed, it could be called into question (Nursing and Midwifery Council 2002, para. 1.2), as the whole picture may not have been considered. While price comparison is the best way to ensure economy, it may not be the only factor to consider. For example, bulk buying may achieve great economies of scale, but buying large amounts of something that has not been used before may prove to be expensive as it may not suit everyone.

Transferability of skills

There appear to be a number of urban myths about learning mathematical skills, and these myths can lead to unwarranted feelings of shame, embarrassment and even fear.

Reflective activity

Cast your mind back to being at school
- List the first three words that come into your mind when you remember being given an abstract mathematical problem to solve
- How did you feel?

Analysing situations such as this may produce feelings of boredom, tedium, dullness and monotony. Many of you may feel your heart sink when you recall the emphasis placed on abstract problems when you were at school. This is why such calculations may be referred to as heart-sink calculations. Many people begin to feel bored, isolated and anxious when presented with problems like this on a regular basis (Ollerton 2003). Ollerton (2003, p. 9) suggests that 'being "made" to do countless exercises and pointless calculations, and made to apply useless formulae' does not encourage anyone to find the answer or to learn how to solve the problem.

There have been many 'top down' strategies over the years to try to change this way of teaching mathematics in order to encourage students to acquire an understanding of and a fascination with mathematics. These strategies have promoted teaching in a way that encourages students to become involved in activities that foster both decision making and problem solving (Ollerton 2003). However, these strategies have not always influenced the way that mathematics is taught in every classroom across the country (House of Commons Committee of Public Accounts 2006). As a result, many working adults seem unable to use the number skills they were taught at school in their everyday work. This is because when you cannot identify with the context of the situation in which the numeracy is set you do not easily engage with the problem, and you do not easily recognise that the skills inherent in problems such as these can be transferred to other similar problems. Indeed, Bransford *et al.* (1989) suggest that this is not unusual and that when most people are confronted with new situations they need help and guidance in order to apply the knowledge and understanding they already have to the new circumstances. Therefore, Chapters 7–10 use a series of patient scenarios which highlight how a variety of numeracy skills are applied in practice.

Teachers' impatience

For many, the mathematical problems presented in class were sometimes very intimidating. Sometimes the speed at which you were expected to calculate the answer was too fast, the teacher's impatience made you flustered, and perhaps if you did the calculation in a different way to the teacher, you were criticised even though you had the correct answer and felt that you could justify what you did. All of these factors may have further compounded any feelings of inadequacy you already had.

If 'heart-sink' calculations and/or a teacher's impatience have ever made you feel like this, you will be gratified to know that Buxton (1981) and Evans (2000), amongst other researchers, suggest that feelings such as these are quite common in working adults. Many theorists conclude that this way of teaching mathematics in schools has left many adults not only disheartened, but also discouraged about their mathematical skills.

World of work/world of nursing

Evidence is now coming forward (Hecht 2002; Hopko *et al.* 2002; Sohn and Doane 2003; Trbovich and LeFevre 2003) that the complexity of some people's work can have a major impact on their thinking processes. This is because the multiple problems that they are working through fill their working memory to such an extent that there is little space left to deal with new problems. Working in complex environments where the decisions you make can have major repercussions on someone's life, and where other members of the team are putting pressure on you to act, means that it may be difficult for you to do mental arithmetic as you have only a small amount of working memory available to you. This reflects the evidence highlighted above in relation to anxiety, working memory and mathematical calculations. Perhaps this is the beginning of evidence to support the intuitive feelings that many nurses have had which Macleod Clark *et al.* (1997) summarised by suggesting that inadequate staffing levels, compounded by a busy ward environment populated with patients with complex problems, inhibits learning.

Moving forward

By now you may have been able to identify a number of factors that produce not only anxiety but also negative coping strategies when you are faced with using your number skills. We will now help you plan to deal with this by identifying some positive coping strategies. If you have identified with any of the anxieties discussed above, the remainder of this chapter will be the next step in your journey to develop your number skills.

Remember that being unable to solve a problem or remember something or making a mistake are not measures of your self-worth. These things happen to everyone from time to time, young or old. You are not a lesser person because of it – such weaknesses reflect your humanity.

Reflective activity

Consider using your Professional Portfolio to capture your learning needs in relation to the factors that may be inhibiting your numeracy skills. You can also record in your portfolio the learning that you achieve by using this book.

Unlocking your potential

If you become anxious when faced with a situation involving calculations, taking all or some of the following actions will help you:

- Take some slow deep breaths
- Have a mantra such as 'I am numerate'
- Consciously refocus your thinking by repeating your mantra to yourself
- Visualise yourself in the resolved situation with the calculation completed successfully
- Use our Skills checklist (see Chapter 3)
- Recognise that this will not be an easy process. It will take time and hard work
- Identify some positive role models
- Remember that differences across men and woman are primarily because people either have a right-dominant brain or a left-dominant brain. It is society that stereotypes the differences into masculine and feminine attributes
- Being aware of stereotype threat improves performance (Aronson *et al.* 2002; Aronson and Williams 2004; Johns *et al.* 2005)
- Remember that differences in performance are seen in both men and women, *not* between men and women
- Remember that everyone makes mistakes from time to time
- Be assured that performance in numeracy is not about your self-worth
- Now start to believe in yourself.

Conclusion

It has been suggested that many people come into nursing because they think that nurses do not do sums. Walkerdine (1998) recognised that this is far from the case when she said 'many occupations traditionally open to women, from nursing to secretarial work, involve considerable calculation'. However, perhaps this is because the numeracy that is inherent in many aspects of nurses' work is not fully appreciated. Indeed, few nurses seem to have given much recognition to the number skills that are in nursing other than those used in medicines and intravenous calculations. This chapter has explored some of the factors that affect either the number skills

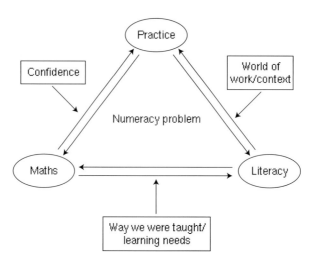

Figure 2.1 *The multidimensional nature of the adult numeracy problem*

of people or their perceptions of their number skills (see Figure 2.1). What it highlights is that difficulties with numeracy are a particularly complex problem, and consequently any solution should address these complexities.

RRRRRRapid recap

Check your progress so far by working through each of the following points
1. What term is used to describe the uncomfortable feelings that many people experience in relation to their numeracy skills?
2. Stereotype threat is said to have an impact on many people's numerical abilities. What kind of effect does it have?
3. List three factors that can affect the ability of adults to calculate
If you have difficulty with more than one of the questions, read through the section again to refresh your understanding before moving on.

References

Allison, S., Beggan, J.K. and Clements, C. (2004) Derogatory stereotypic beliefs and evaluations of male nurses. *Equal Opportunities International*, **23**(3/4/5), 162–178.

Aronson, J. (2004) The threat of stereotype. *Educational Leadership*, **62**(3) 14–20.

Aronson, J., Lustina, M.J., Good, C., Keough, K., Steele, C.M., Brown J. (1999) When white men can't do math: necessary and sufficient factors in stereotype threat. *Journal of Experimental Social Psychology*, **35**, 29–46.

Ashcraft, M.H. (2002) Math anxiety: personal, educational, and cognitive consequences. *Current Directions in Psychological Science*, **11**(5), 181–185.

Ashcraft, M.H. and Kirk, E.P. (2001) The relationship among working memory, math anxiety, and performance. *Journal of Experimental Psychology; General*, **130**, 224–237.

Ashcraft, M.H., Kirk, E.P. and Hopko, D. (1998) On the cognitive consequences of mathematics anxiety. In: Donlan, C. (ed) *The Development of Mathematical Skills*. Psychology Press, Hove.

Baron-Cohen, S. (2004) *The Essential Difference*. Penguin, London.

Bar-Tal, Y. and Guinote, A. (2002) Who exhibits more stereotypical thinking? The effect of need and ability to achieve cognitive structure on stereotyping. *European Journal of Personality*, **16**, 313–331.

Bloom, A. (1968) The republic of Plato. In Consuming images: How television commercials that elicit stereotype threat can restrain women academically and professionally. Davies, P.G., Spencer, S.J., Quinn, D.M. and Gerhardstein, R.(2002). *Personality and Social Psychology Bulletin*, **28**(12) 1615–1628.

Bransford, J.D., Franks, J.J., Vye, N.J. and Sherwood, R.D. (1989) New approaches to instruction: because wisdom can't be told. In: *Similarity and Analogical Reasoning* (eds Vosniadou, S. and Ortony, A.). Cambridge University Press, Cambridge and New York.

Buxton, L. (1981) *Do you panic about maths? Coping with maths anxiety*. Heinemann Educational, London.

Cadinu, M., Maass, A., Frigerio, S., Impagliazzo, L., and Latinotti, S. (2003) Stereotype threat: The effect of expectancy on performance. *European Journal of Social Psychology*, **33**, 267–285.

Clarke, J. and O'Neill, C.S. (2001) An analysis of how the *Irish Times* portrayed Irish nursing during the 1999 strike. *Nursing Ethics*, **8**(4), 350–359.

Concise Oxford Dictionary (2005) (11th edn) Oxford University Press, Oxford.

Davies, C. (1998) *Gender and the Professional Predicament in Nursing*. Open University Press, Buckingham.

Davies, P.G., Spencer, S.J., Quinn, D.M. and Gerhardstein, R. (2002) Consuming images: How television commercials that elicit stereotype threat can restrain women academically and professionally. *Personality and Social Psychology Bulletin*, **28**(12), 1615–1628.

Evans, J. (2000) *Adult's Mathematical Thinking and Emotions: a Study of Numerate Practices*. Taylor & Francis, London.

Foels, R. and Pappas, C.J. (2004) Learning and unlearning the myths we are taught: Gender and social dominance orientation. *Sex Roles*, **50**(11/12), June.

Ford, T.E., Ferguson, M.A., Brooks J.K. and Hagadone, K.M. (2004) Coping sense of humour reduces effects of stereotype threat on women's math performance. *Personality and Social Psychology Bulletin*, **30**(5), 643–653.

Goldenberg, S (2005) Why women are poor at science, by Harvard president. www.guardian.co.uk/life/science/story/0,12996,1392806,00.html.

Hecht, S.A. (2002) Counting on working memory in simple arithmetic when counting is used for problem solving. *Memory & Cognition*, **30**(3), 447–455.

Heskins, F.M. (1997) Exploring dichotomies of caring, gender and technology in intensive care nursing: A qualitative approach. *Intensive and Critical Care Nursing*, **13**, 65–71.

Hopko, D.R., McNeil, D.W., Lejuez, C.W., Ashcraft M.H., Eifert, G.H. and Riel J. (2003) The effects of anxious responding on mental arithmetic and lexical decision task performance. *Anxiety Disorders*, **17**, 647–665.

House of Commons Committee of Public Accounts (2006) *Skills for Life: Improving Adult Literacy and Numeracy*. 21st report of Session 2005–06. The Stationery Office Ltd, London.

Johns, M., Schmader, T. and Martens, A. (2005) Knowing is half the battle: Teaching stereotype threat as a means of improving women's math performance. *Psychological Science*, **16**(3), 175–179.

Kendrick, K. (2005) The Left, Right and Centre of Male and Female Brain Politics. Transcript of a lecture given at Gresham College on 22/10/05. www.gresham.ac.uk/event.asp?PageId=45&EventId=369.

Keonig, A.M. and Eagly, A.H. (2005) Stereotype threat in men on a test of social sensitivity. *Sex Roles*, **52**(7/8), 489–496.

Macleod Clark, J., Maben, J. and Jones, K. (1997) Project 2000: shifting perceptions of the philosophy and practice of nursing. *Journal of Advanced Nursing*, **26**(9), 246–256.

McIntyre, R.B., Lord, C.G., Gresky, D.M., Ten Eyck L.L., Jay Frye, G.D. and Bond Jr., C.F. (2005) A social impact trend in the effects of role models on alleviating women's mathematics stereotype threat. *Current Research in Social Psychology*, **10**(9), 116–136.

Niven, N. (2000) *Health Psychology for Health Care Professionals*. Churchill Livingstone, Edinburgh.

Nursing and Midwifery Council (2002) *Code of Professional Conduct*. Nursing and Midwifery Council, London.

Nursing and Midwifery Council (2005) Statistical analysis of the register, 1 April 2004–31 March 2005. www.nmc-uk.org.uk.

Ollerton, M. (2003) *Getting the Buggers to Add Up*. Continuum, London.

Pert, C. (1999) *Molecules of Emotion*. Pocket Books, London.

Reverby, S. (1987) A caring dilemma: Womanhood and nursing in historical perspective. *Nursing Research*, **36**, 1–5.

Rittle Johnson, B. and Siegler, R.S. (1998) The relationship between conceptual and procedural knowledge in learning mathematics. In: *The Development of Mathematical Skills* (ed. Donlan, C.). Psychology Press, Hove.

Schmader, T., Johns, M. and Barquissau, M. (2004) The costs of accepting gender differences: The role of stereotype endorsement in women's experience in the math domain. *Sex Roles*, **50**(11/12), 835–850.

Shepherd, J. (2006) *Tutors in despair at illiterate freshers. The Times Higher Education Supplement*, 10 February. www.thes.co.uk.

Sichtermann, B. (1986) *Femininity: the politics of the personal* (translated by John Whitlam). Polity, Cambridge.

Smith, J.K., and White, P.H. (2002) An examination of implicitly activated, explicitly activated, and nullified stereotypes on mathematical performance: It is not just a woman's issue. *Sex Roles*, **48**(12/13), 179–187.

Sohn, Y.W. and Doane, S.M. (2003) Roles of working memory capacity and long-term working memory skill in complex task performance. *Memory & Cognition*, **31**(3), 458–466.

Taylor, E.W. (2001) Transformative learning theory: A neurobiological perspective of the role of emotions and unconscious ways of knowing. *International Journal of Lifelong Education*, **20**(3), 218–236.

Tickle tests, http://web.tickle.com/tests/brain/index_main.jsp.

Trbovich, P.L. and LeFevre, J.A. (2003) Phonological and visual working memory in mental addition. *Memory & Cognition*, **31**(5), 738–745.

Walkerdine, V. (1998) *Counting girls out: girls and mathematics*. Falmer Press, London.

Warelow, P.J. (1996) Is caring the ethical ideal? *Journal of Advanced Nursing*, **24**, 655–661.

White, K. (2002) Nursing as vocation. *Nursing Ethics*, **9**(3), 279–290.

Whittock, M. and Leonard, L. (2003) Stepping outside the stereotype: A pilot study of the motivations and experiences of males in the nursing profession. *Journal of Nursing Management*, **11**, 242–249.

Women and Work Commission (2006) *Shaping a Fairer Future*. www.womenand equalityunit.gov.uk/women_work_commisison

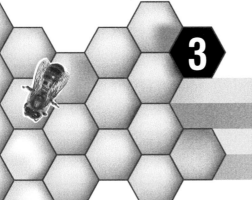

3

From problem to solution, identifying the process and introducing some tools

Learning outcomes

By the end of this chapter you should be able to:

- Identify common problem areas when using number skills in nursing practice

- Explore strategies for learning number skills

- Identify a problem-solving approach to solve practice calculations

- Identify the individual skills within number calculations

- Recognise personal strengths and areas for further development

In Chapter 2 we established that nurses and other health care professionals have been identified as having varying degrees of difficulty with numeracy. It is important to reiterate here that numeracy skills are problematic for the population as a whole.

Pólya (1990), one of the gurus of mathematics education, struggled to understand why, despite his best teaching efforts, his students did not seem to understand or master what they were taught. His concerns centred on his experience that, even when students had been exposed to similar teaching and learning strategies on previous occasions, they did not appear to be able to *transfer* this to new situations. Pólya developed a strategy to enable his students to learn from their previous experiences. His strategy started with asking his students to consider the problem.

This links well to contemporary approaches used in nurse education. Many pre-registration programmes have adopted a problem-based learning strategy. This approach uses situations or scenarios that are context related, meaning that they are examples generated from practice. This is important when trying to address numeracy skills. Much of the literature (Ollerton 2003) suggests that students do not learn abstract concepts effectively, but that these become much more meaningful when they are clearly related to the student's own world of work. Another strength of this approach is that the student identifies their own individual learning needs. Bath and Blais (1993) suggest that learning numeracy skills in a way that reinforces the student's preferred learning style is more successful.

Problem-based learning

Problem-based learning is an approach used, for example, in medical education as it generates problems from real-life situations that the students need to understand and solve. Many nursing curricula have adopted this approach but have dropped the word 'problem' because nursing activities are related to patient needs as well as problems; they thus refer to this approach as 'enquiry-based learning'. The student gets involved in their own learning by identifying what they do not know, and then finding out the information. One of the strengths of this approach is that students 'develop skills in critical thinking, analysis, reflection and evaluation' (Ashby *et al.* 2005, p. 22). It is suggested that this approach enhances transferability of skills; indeed, the students in the Nottingham evaluative study themselves commented that it helped them to link theory to practice (Ashby *et al.* 2005). Barnard *et al.* (2005) suggest that courses that have enquiry as the main strategy have problem solving as the focus and foster critical thinking.

The first step, therefore, is exploring the problem. This is a useful strategy for students of nursing to engage in as it is closely linked to the nursing process and its stages of assessment, planning, implementation and evaluation. As part of the nursing process, the nurse collects information about the patient by asking questions about them or their relatives, recording observations, reading case notes, etc. (assessment). The nurse then identifies the nursing care the patient requires, taking into account interventions, staff and equipment needed (planning); carries out the care (implementation); and finally reviews how successful the nursing interventions were (evaluation). Identifying and exploring the problem in this way leads us to solutions or outcomes – it is problem solving. Price (2003, p. 47) supports this, stating that 'problem solving is . . . central to caring for patients'.

Problem solving

Problem solving can also be described as information processing, the aim of which is to assist the decision-making process. While this is a useful process when considering desired patient outcomes and therefore the most appropriate nursing interventions, we can also transfer this process to learning. If we want to use problem solving in other situations, i.e. learning, we would still go through the stages of recognising the problem, considering a range of strategies, and taking the most appropriate action having considered the alternatives. This process is based on the assumption that we bring to the problem some previous knowledge, e.g. our experience of similar problems (Price 2003). The link between numeracy and problem solving may not be immediately obvious. Arnold (1998) suggests that in some situations, e.g. fluid balance calculations, the problem was not with nurses' numeracy skills, but in identifying the problem to be solved. For example, think about *how* you would answer the following questions.

Over to you

Refresher – identifying the problem

a. How many different ways can you multiply two whole positive numbers together to make 32? Identify these

b. How many different pairs of whole positive numbers add up to 12? Identify these.

Can you identify the process you went through to answer the questions above? Ollerton (2003, p. 102) suggests that 'mathematics is essentially . . . a set of tools for solving problems, students need to experience mathematics in problem solving ways'. He suggests that the questions asked in the refresher above pose problems, and therefore involve the student in problem solving. Therefore, the first step has to be identifying the problem/what is to be investigated.

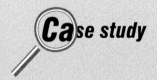

Case study

Attending a slimming club

Consider the following scenario: You decide to try to lose a few pounds by joining a local slimming group. However, it is a while since you have been weighed. You are really concerned with the target weight loss your club leader has identified for you, as 5 kilograms seems a lot, even though it is suggested you do this slowly. Before the meeting you thought you had about 3/4 stone to lose.

Everyone else at the club meeting seems to be very familiar with kg and recommended weight ranges, so you resolve to be better informed yourself for the next meeting, as you suddenly feel a little foolish.

Problem solving is an essential skill for today's nurses, but like any other skill it needs to be learnt, and sometimes we need cues or prompts to help us get started. These cues are often questions, so you might find applying the following questions to the scenario outlined above a useful place to start.

The problem:

1. Do you understand what you have been asked to do?
2. Have you done this before?
3. How did you do it then?

Applying question 1 to the above scenario, you need to:

- Identify the appropriate weight for your age, gender and height
- Find out how kilograms and stones compare
- Convert stones into kilograms (this may involve changing the stones into pounds first)
- Compare your goal weight with your current weight.

Only you can answer questions 2 and 3, but one of the most effective ways of learning is to use your experience; it can help to develop independent thinking.

Learning from experience (experiential learning)

Experiential learning is a continuous process of creating new knowledge by reflecting on experience (Sewchuk 2005). For example, if we are comparing prices and trying to establish whether it was cheaper to buy our favourite shampoo at the high-street chemist who is offering three for two on bottles of 200 ml, or to pop to the local supermarket and buy a large bottle of 500 ml, we would need to work out the *unit* price. In other words it would be useful to compare the cost of 100 ml. If our calculation shows that the cost of 100 ml is £15, our experience would tell us that £15 was too much for our usual shampoo, and we would therefore adjust our calculation and assume the price to be £1·50.

You may have been doing this informally, but in order to use this strategy effectively, you may need to use some cues/questions. There are several models available to help you do this. Most of these experiential models use a framework based upon exploring the experience. We start by remembering what happened during the experience, thinking about what was happening, and identifying what we felt in order to identify where the gaps in our knowledge are. In order to use them again, we need to identify the learning strategies that were helpful to us. We also need to test out these theories by using them in the next experience. This process is often described as a cycle (Kolb 1984), as having had the second experience the whole process starts again, thus establishing a continuous process of refining our learning strategies. An important aspect of the process is understanding what helps us to learn effectively. You may need some help to guide you through this experiential process initially, either from a skilled colleague/ facilitator or a text. You may find the following chapters useful: 'What is reflective practice?' and 'Knowing ourselves' in Jasper (2003) *Beginning Reflective Practice*.

Having considered the problem raised in the scenario on p. 36 and identified what information you need in order to understand how to convert pounds into kilograms, you then need to carry out the conversion and compare your answer with recommended weights. These weights are based upon height, age and gender. To do this you need to go through the following stages.

> ## Over to you
>
> 1. Identify sources of information
> 2. Identify the sequence of the calculation (BODMAS)
> 3. Consider if you know a *formula* that might help.

1. It is not necessary for us to carry information like conversions in our heads. In practice, most health professionals would refer to a chart. However, it is really important to have a *valid* source to help us with this calculation. Many nurses in clinical areas often use information they have copied from a colleague, and are unaware of the source of this information so are unable to check whether it is accurate or reliable. Also, the more often a piece of information is copied, the more chances there are for it to be copied inaccurately

2. If we are involved in a calculation that requires more than one operation to reach the answer, e.g. multiplication and subtraction in our scenario, there is a correct order in which to carry out these separate operations. This is referred to as BODMAS, which is the abbreviation for Brackets, pOwers/roots, Division, Multiplication, Addition and Subtraction (Kearsley Bullen 2003). If you are not familiar with this, in Chapter 4, p. 61 there is an explanation and some worked examples

3. There are several examples of formulae which can help us arrive at the right answer, e.g. when calculating intravenous drip rates. Again, these are identified in Chapter 4 and worked examples are provided. This chapter is concerned with *how* we can become confident in learning how to calculate; Chapter 4 will provide you with the tools.

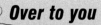

Over to you

Arriving at the answer

1. Try to 'guestimate' the answer
2. Carry out the calculation
3. State the answer in the correct form (e.g. SI units – this term is explained in Chapter 5)
4. *Round up* figures if necessary.

1. One of the most difficult situations to be in is where we are asked to provide an answer to a situation of which we have no experience, and therefore cannot visualise. If you were asked to calculate an intravenous drip rate without having seen an intravenous infusion, you would probably produce an inaccurate and improbable answer without realising it. However, if you have seen an intravenous infusion in progress, noted the smallness of the drop, perhaps seen a colleague timing the drip rate using a watch, you would be able to assume that 6·4 or 640 drops per minute would be almost impossible to count. We are therefore using previous experience, and even part of the problem-solving process, to reject improbable answers. It is a useful strategy therefore to have a rough idea in our head (a guestimate) of what would be a reasonable answer. Most experienced nurses, for example, know that if the patient is to have 3 litres of a fluid in 24 hours via infusion, the drip rate will be approximately 40 drops per minute. However, this should always be calculated (intravenous-giving sets vary in how many drops per ml they deliver) and not relied upon, but it does offer a baseline for comparison. This is discussed further in Chapter 4

2. To carry out the calculation we need to feel comfortable about our skills in this area. When we are involved in a calculation in the clinical area we need to be sure we are safe. If we are unsure about our skills it may limit our ability to function in clinical areas. More commonly though, we may over-rely on other people to calculate for us, particularly when working with more senior colleagues. We have no way of knowing how effective their numeracy skills are, and as accountable employees we need to reassure ourselves that the correct answer is identified in relation to any calculation. One problem inherent in the calculation of doses of medicines is that we do the calculations occasionally. If we did them every day, they would quickly become second nature.

Consider also that in most clinical areas, because of pressures of work, nurses often carry out medicine rounds on their own. They therefore need to be confident about their numeracy skills base, just as they are about their other skills. Duthie (1988) and the Nursing and Midwifery Council (2004) recommend that wherever there is a calculation involved, two nurses should take part

3. The example of the intravenous infusion rate above (40 drops per minute) involves two measurements: volume (drops) and time. Volume is measured using SI units. Volume and time are discussed in Chapter 5

4. We also need to ensure that we can *use* the answer we have obtained. Does if feel right? Have we been involved in this kind calculation before? Did we have a rough estimate before we started to compare our answer with?

Over to you

Confirming the answer

1. When you have identified your answer, compare it to your estimate. Does the answer seem reasonable?
2. How do you feel about the process? Was it easier or more difficult than you expected?
3. Can you identify which parts of the calculation process you were comfortable with, and which you need more help with?
4. How will you develop your skills?

This final *Over to you* is compatible with the evaluation process both of the nursing care plan and experiential learning. What was the outcome? Was it appropriate, i.e. did we achieve what we set out to achieve? What will we do again? What do we need to change? This is also compatible with the reflective process, and it is important that it reflects how we felt and what our strengths are. It then takes us on to the next step – if we have identified weaknesses, how will we overcome them?

Reflection is becoming more and more important in nursing. It enables us to learn from our experience and therefore it is as a key component of experiential learning. One reason for its current popularity as a learning strategy in nursing is that it does *allow* us to explore our feelings. Also it helps us to make sense of the often bewildering world of practice (Jasper 2003; Chapelhow *et al.* 2005).

Hopefully these questions will kick-start your thinking process, and if used regularly will become very familiar so that you do not even need to go through the individual steps. Those of you with some nursing experience will perhaps have already recognised this process as being similar to the nursing process – assessment, planning, implementation and evaluation.

Pólya (1990) describes these processes as **heuristic**. He also believes in the importance of learning from personal experience. In order for the learner to master numeracy he identifies the stages of:

- Understanding the problem
- Using experience from related problems to plan
- Carrying out the plan
- Asking yourself whether you really believe the answer you have got.

We have taken these similar approaches and distilled them into a tool that you can use (Table 3.1).

We have tried to identify a process that you can use whenever you meet numbers and calculations in your practice. Along the way we have introduced a lot of terminology: BODMAS, formula, calculation, SI units, 'rounding up' figures. Chapters 4 and 5 revisit these and explain what the terms refer to and how they should be used. You will then be able to use the process outlined above.

Keywords

Heuristic

Refers to approaches to learning that enable someone to discover, and to methods which encourage learners to find out for themselves

---

Reflective activity

Think about what you have just read

1. How do you feel about the ideas that have been expressed?
2. How familiar are you with terminology we have just introduced?
3. Do you have an understanding of kilograms, or are you more comfortable when weight is expressed in stones and pounds?
4. Are you able to convert from one unit to the other?

You need to answer these questions honestly so that you can use the rest of this book effectively.

Table 3.1 Comparing approaches

Nursing process stages	Pólya's strategies	Our tool (Skills checklist)
Assess	Understand the problem	What am I being asked to do?
Plan	Use previous experience to plan	Identify number principles and formulae
Implement	Carry out the plan	Apply the number principles and perform the calculation, stating the answer appropriately
Evaluate (and modify)	How believable is the answer?	Is it a correct answer? How do I feel about the process? What do I need to do now?

Building confidence by reinforcing what skills we possess

We want to reassure you about the skills you already possess, so we will begin by using what we refer to as life examples.

Pursuing the example in the scenario on page 36, you have established that you have 5 kilograms to lose. There are several diets that you could choose, but all of them involve some kind of calculation.

Some well-known and established slimming groups use a system of points based upon the fat content and calorific value of foods, so comparing two different entities to calculate points. The number of points that an individual needs to consume per day is based on the ideal weight for their height, gender and age, but also how much weight they need to lose.

However, low-carbohydrate diets are based upon the carbohydrate content of foods, which is identified on the label. Sometimes the diet is only concerned with the carbohydrate content; those which have a high carbohydrate content should be avoided. To complicate matters, some diets refer to 'net carbs', which are obtained by deducting the amount of fibre from the amount of carbohydrate. The label often identifies the type of carbohydrates, for example sugars and sweeteners. Most diet products are artificially sweetened and so the sweetener may or may not count. Polyols are an artificial sweetener which does not have to be counted. This type of diet only requires the use of subtraction.

This is further complicated by the GI diet, which also focuses on the carbohydrate value of foods, but takes it a stage further and considers the glycaemic index. The carbohydrates are classified in terms of how long they take to reach the bloodstream (the glycaemic index, or GI). Those carbohydrates which are absorbed slowly are considered to be less problematic, and so are allowed in larger quantities.

There is also a glycaemic load (GL) diet, which considers the glycaemic index and portion control. If the label states that there are 20 grams of carbohydrate in 100 grams of the product, and the diet guidelines suggest we should only consume 15 grams of this food group, we need to calculate how many grams of carbohydrate are in this product in order to make sure we consume no more than the recommended intake. This involves division and multiplication as well as addition and subtraction.

Reflective activity

Take a moment to consider what numeracy skills you used yesterday. Did you calculate your calorie or carbohydrate intake? Did you buy some groceries? In which case, were you able to roughly anticipate what the bill would be, and identify the change you needed? Did you calculate a bus fare or the cost of a round of drinks?

These calculations can be straightforward, e.g. a bus fare, or complex, e.g. a round of drinks, groceries. They involve the skills of addition and subtraction, and possibly even division if we are working out our individual contribution to the drinks kitty. Not only are you able to carry out this kind of calculation, but you are able to carry it out in a different situation, which means you can transfer the skills. If we were to list more examples, such as placing a bet, comparing costs between the different mobile phone providers (monthly rental, call tariff, etc.), it should become more obvious to you that you already possess some number/numeracy skills that might involve complex calculations. There are likely to be some others that you are not as comfortable with.

Addition, subtraction, multiplication and division are the four *basic* types of calculation that contribute to the more complex calculation that we undertake. They are described as the *four rules of arithmetic* (Kearsley Bullen 2003; Coben and Atere-Roberts 2005). It is important that you are confident in these skills before you tackle the clinical examples.

Identifying those skills which need developing

Have a go at the calculations identified below. Check your answers (Appendix C) so that you get an indication of where your strengths and weaknesses (if any) are. We advise you to revisit these same calculations at regular intervals to identify the progress you are making in your ability to calculate successfully, and the impact that has upon your confidence.

> ## Over to you
>
> **Refresher – arithmetic**
>
> Addition
> a. $56 + 8 =$
> b. $561 + 18 =$
> c. $56 \cdot 1 + 10 =$
> d. $56 \cdot 1 + 1 \cdot 8 =$
> e. $56 \cdot 1 + 1 \cdot 8 + 19 + 0 \cdot 1 =$
>
> Subtraction
> a. $56 - 8 =$
> b. $561 - 18 =$
> c. $56 \cdot 1 - 10 =$
> d. $56 \cdot 1 - 1 \cdot 8 =$
> e. $56 \cdot 1 - 9 \cdot 5 - 48 =$
>
> Multiplication
> a. $56 \times 8 =$
> b. $561 \times 18 =$
> c. $56 \cdot 1 \times 10 =$
> d. $56 \cdot 1 \times 1 \cdot 8 =$
> e. $56 \times 8 \times 10 =$
>
> Division
> a. $56 \div 8 =$
> b. $561 \div 18 =$
> c. $56 \cdot 1 \div 10 =$
> d. $56 \cdot 1 \div 1 \cdot 8 =$
> e. $56 \div 8 \div 1 \cdot 4 =$
>
> And all together . . .
> a. $561 + 8 - 1 \cdot 8 \times 10 \div 1 \cdot 4 =$
> b. $561 + 8 - (18 \times 10) =$

Check your answers with those given below.

Addition

a. 64

b. 579

c. 66·1

d. 57·9

e. 77

Subtraction

a. 48

b. 543

c. 46·1

d. 54·3

e. −1·4

Multiplication

a. 448

b. 10,098

c. 561

d. 100·98

e. 4,480

Division

a. 7

b. 31·1666. . .

c. 5·61

d. 31·1666. . .

e. 5

And all together . . .

a. 556·143

b. 389

Having undertaken these examples, you need to think about how you felt about them as well as how successful you were. We suggest that you return to these calculations on a regular basis in order to review and record your progress. We have collected the arithmetic refreshers together in Appendix B for you to use. Being able to see that your numeracy skills are improving is a great motivator.

You need some strategies for success. The first step is for you to understand where your strengths are, but also to identify those areas you need to develop, so ask yourself the following questions.

Reflective activity

1. How did you feel about undertaking the refresher above?
2. Did you understand what you were being asked to do?
3. What method did you choose to work out these examples – did you do it in your head, with a pencil and paper, did you use a calculator?
4. Did you estimate an answer first, to test your final answer?
5. Did you use some method/formula to work out the answers?
6. Have you met problems like this in a work context?
7. Which of these did you find easy and which difficult (if any)?
8. How will you address these difficulties?

(See Coben & Atere-Roberts (2005), Pólya (1990))

If you have answered 'no' to questions 2, 4, 5 and 6, be reassured that many of your colleagues, if asked, probably feel the same way. The possible reasons for this have been discussed in Chapter 2. However, we want to improve both your competence and your confidence. In order to make best use of the chapters that follow, it is important for you to identify why you have problems in specific areas. Blais and Bath (1992) identified that nurses' difficulties with calculation could be due to conceptual difficulties rather than problems using numbers. They suggested that nurses had difficulty in 'setting up the problem', in other words, they did not understand what they were being asked to do. Consider your answers to the above questions as you work your way through Chapters 4 and 5, as this will enable you to capitalise on those strategies best suited to your learning needs.

Conclusions

This chapter has discussed how complex the process of learning numeracy skills is. We have identified that the skills involved are the same skills used in any other aspect of learning about nursing. There are rules inherent in undertaking calculations and these are explored in later chapters. We have also offered a basic arithmetic refresher based upon the *four rules of arithmetic* to help you determine your strengths and areas that need developing.

RRRRRRapid recap

Check your progress so far by working through each of the following points
1. What are the *four rules of arithmetic*?
2. Identify some number systems which you can use in calculations
3. Identify Pólya's strategies for solving mathematical problems
4. Identify some learning strategies which relate to understanding and learning numbers

If you have difficulty with more than one of the questions, read through the appropriate section again to refresh your understanding before moving on.

References

Arnold, G. (1998) Refinements in the dimensional analysis of dose calculation problem-solving. *Nurse Educator*, **23**(3), 22–26.

Ashby, J., Hubbert V., Cotrel-Gibbons, L., Cox, K., Digan, J., Lewis, K., Langmack, G., *et al.* (2005) The enquiry based learning experience: An evaluation project. *Nurse Education in Practice*, **6**(1), 22–30.

Barnard, A., Nash, R. and O'Brien, M. (2005) Information literacy: Developing lifelong skills through nursing education. *Journal of Nursing Education*, **44**(11), 505–511.

Bath, J.B. and Blais, K. (1993) Learning style as a predictor of drug dosage ability. *Nurse Educator*, **18** (1), 33–36.

Blais, K. and Bath, J.B. (1992) Drug calculation errors of baccalaureate nursing students. *Nurse Education*, **17**, 12–15.

Chapelhow, C., Crouch, S., Fisher, M. and Walsh, A. (2005) *Uncovering Skills for Practice*. Nelson Thornes, Cheltenham.

Coben, D. and Atere-Roberts, E. (2005) *Calculations for Nursing and Healthcare*, 2nd edn. Palgrave Macmillan, Hampshire.

Duthie, R.B. (1988) *Department of Health Guidelines for the Safe and Secure Handling of Medicines*. Department of Health, London.

Jasper, M. (2003) *Beginning Reflective Practice*. Nelson Thornes, Cheltenham.

Kearsley Bullen, R. (2003) *BBC KS3 Bitesize Revision*. BBC Worldwide, England. See also www.bbc.co.uk/bitesize.

Kolb, D.A. (1984) *Experiential Learning: Experience as the Source of Learning and Development*. Prentice Hall, Englewood Cliffs, NJ.

Nursing and Midwifery Council (2004) *Guidelines for the Administration of Medicines*. NMC, London.

Ollerton, M. (2003) *Getting the Buggers to Add Up*. Continuum, London.

Pólya, G. (1990) *How to Solve it: a New Aspect of Mathematical Method*, 2nd edn. Penguin, London.

Price, B. (2003) Understanding the origins of practice problems. *Nursing Standard* **17**(50), 47–53.

Sewchuk, D.H. (2005) Experiential learning – a theoretical framework for perioperative education. *Association of Operating Room Nurses. AORN Journal* **81**(6), 1311–1318.

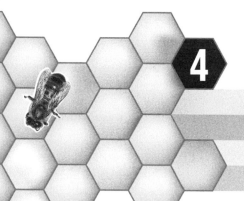

Understanding and using numbers

In Chapter 3 we suggested that it is important to identify how we can learn to calculate based upon our individual needs and using a logical approach that acknowledges prior learning. Our approach follows that of Pólya (1990), who identified a set of heuristic strategies to help his students. His strategies are a set of general problem-solving techniques, which he suggested mathematicians used frequently but rarely acknowledged. Pólya was an internationally renowned mathematician and we cannot compare this book to his work, although the aim of both is to help students.

Pólya outlined four strategies that would help his students focus their thinking. These were identified above (in Chapter 3) as being:

1. Understand the problem
2. Try to use experience from related problems to devise a plan
3. Carry out the plan (checking each step as you go)
4. Examine the solution (ask yourself if you really believe the answer you got).

The first step therefore is to understand the problem.

We need to understand calculations and numbers in order to understand the problem. Ollerton (2003, p. 102) contends that mathematics is 'essentially a collection of ideas . . . and a set of tools for solving problems'. This chapter provides an overview of number systems, number and perception, and formulae related to nursing practice.

Worked examples of basic calculations

It is necessary in a book such as this to provide the reader with an overview of basic calculations, a *refresher*. We started this process in Chapter 3, by getting you to identify some strengths and weaknesses in basic arithmetic.

We also need to provide a review of the calculations frequently used in nursing practice. This will include explanations of how to perform the calculations and also calculations for you to try (answers are provided at the back of the book). We have already identified the need to apply numeracy to the real world of work.

There is a sound rationale for this calculation review. Firstly, it serves as a reminder for those of you who have not undertaken calculations in a formal way for some time. Secondly, it provides you with a baseline of how you performed the first time in order for you to compare your progress after reading the book. Undertaking calculations yourself (performing a diagnostic test) to help you identify your strengths and weaknesses has been shown to be a successful strategy for student nurses (Hutton 1998). Providing you with diagnostic tests throughout will help to build your confidence and you will want to move on to more demanding calculations (Knight 2001).

This is an important step for you to take, but Chapter 2 has outlined some of the reasons why, at this moment, you may have a strong temptation to put the book down or turn to a different chapter. If you move on to the practice-based examples in Chapters 7–10 without reminding yourself of the basic calculations of addition, subtraction, multiplication and division, you may start to feel very uncomfortable with the calculations in the scenarios.

You may already be confident about your skills, which is absolutely fine, but we have tried to take a different approach – so you might want to linger a while.

Much of the educational literature makes a clear case that learning should be seen as useful for the student (hence the patient case studies generated from practice) and that it should be enjoyable (Ollerton 2003). Although it might be difficult to persuade you that learning about numbers and calculation can be enjoyable, there seems to be a growing enthusiasm for a number puzzle called Su Doku. In fact *The Times* has published a book which says: 'Su Doku . . . comes with a health warning: it is seriously addictive' (*The Times* 2005). Ollerton (2003) suggests that we enjoy this type of activity because we derive pleasure from the challenge of solving logic puzzles such as this, and that we can apply this kind of problem-solving approach to numeracy problems. So to get you started we have provided three examples of Su Doku, rated easy to difficult.

The Times (2005) describes Su Doku as a 'number-placing puzzle', which is apt as all it involves is placing the numbers 1 to 9 in particular sequences. The standard puzzle contains a box of 81 squares, nine across and nine down. Within this box there are smaller grids of nine squares, so each large box contains nine grids, three across and three down.

The principle is that you place the numbers 1 to 9 into each grid of nine squares (some numbers are provided for you), but each line in the bigger box (both across and down) should also contain the numbers 1 to 9, for example

1	2	3	4	5	6	7	8	9
9	4	7						
8	6	5						
7								
6								
5								
4								
3								
2								

Most Su Doku puzzle books identify strategies that you can employ to solve the puzzle. For example:

- It is easier to identify where to place numbers when a lot of the numbers already appear; if the puzzle contains a lot of 4s but not a lot of 1s, the fewer missing 4s are easier to place
- If a line contains several completed squares this would be a good place to start, likewise if a grid contains several completed squares this might be a good place to start. This would depend on what numbers appear, and the numbers in nearby lines or grids
- You could also try to place individual numbers in each grid rather than trying to complete lines or grids, for example placing a 3 in each grid.

In reality it is a combination of strategies that work, and having the patience to keep going! The Su Doku puzzle books on sale contain much more comprehensive strategies for the completion of these puzzles.

See the following examples.

Original grid

	1	2	6	8			9	
6					4		1	
8		5	2			3	7	
					7	5	2	3
			4		6			
3	8	1	9					
	5	4			2	8		1
	7		3					2
	3			5	9	7	6	

Original grid

Completed grid

7	1	2	6	8	3	4	9	5
6	9	3	5	7	4	2	1	8
8	4	5	2	9	1	3	7	6
4	6	9	8	1	7	5	2	3
5	2	7	4	3	6	1	8	9
3	8	1	9	2	5	6	4	7
9	5	4	7	6	2	8	3	1
1	7	6	3	4	8	9	5	2
2	3	8	1	5	9	7	6	4

Completed grid

Now try these puzzles.

1. The 'easy' puzzle

		7	9		4	6		
	1	2	3		8	9	7	
	5		2	4	6		9	
2		4		9		5		7
	9		7	8	5		2	
	6	9	5		7	2	4	
		5			9	3		

2. The 'medium' puzzle

								6
			4	1				
					3	1	4	
	9					6	7	
	7				9	5		
		3		7	1		9	2
		9	6	4			8	3
		6	2		8	4	1	
4					5	9		

3. The 'difficult' puzzle

			6					
5					7		2	
	8			4	9			
				6	2	7	5	
	9	5				4	8	
7							9	
4	1			3				
	6	7		5		3		
		8	2				6	

The answers to these puzzles can be found at the back of the book.

The Su Doku puzzles have not involved you in any calculation, but you have been engaged in number recognition and placing, which has involved the use of logic. We know that a number can only appear once in any box or line. Logic is about relationships and/or interactions between facts, and so is often used in **empirical** (scientific) studies to predict or explain results. For example, if we know that a lot of medications routinely used in a specific clinical area can cause nausea, then if a patient suddenly starts to complain of feeling sick, a logical action to take would be to check the patient's medication sheet. However, skilled nurses often use their experience to explain why patients are reacting in a particular way, and this is based upon a holistic assessment of the patient. So logic would be only a part of this, and some would argue that logic does not help us explain the complex care currently delivered. More recently the concept of logic has been linked to effective decision making, particularly in the context of good decisions related to the evidence base for practice (Dowding and Thompson 2003). So whatever nursing problem we are faced with, examining it and applying logic is a good place to start. This is a useful strategy for tackling number problems and can help us identify appropriate rules and/or formulae to use. This process can be described as deductive, in that it takes the learner through a set of formal rules to a logical conclusion based upon processes of problem solving (Sierpinska 1994).

⊙━ Keywords

Empirical
Generally used in nursing to refer to knowledge that is obtained through scientific experiment. In other words, empirical knowledge can be proved. Carper (1978) describes this as one way 'of knowing' in her discussion of the types of knowledge that help us understand nursing.

o—r *Keywords*

....

Variables

Used to describe a number of
different explanations or values

Sometimes, when completing this kind of logic problem, our eyes
seem to work faster than our brain and the number to complete
the grid pops into our head before we have worked through the
variables logically. We seem to see the answer. This might be
explained by the fact that we are using previous experience or are
unconsciously working it out in our head.

This might be explained by our individual learning style. Chinn
(1998) has an interesting way of explaining this. He refers to
'inchworms' and 'grasshoppers'. Inchworms are logical, taking things
a step at a time, using mathematical formulae to help them find
answers. Grasshoppers like to go straight to the answer; they see the
whole picture and are good at mental arithmetic. Chinn goes on to
suggest that grasshoppers like to estimate, and often obtain the right
answer without 'knowing how they got there'. Neither way is right,
but both have strengths. They also have weaknesses, and we do need
to be able to reassure ourselves that the answers we reach are the
correct ones.

Grasshoppers, because they see the whole, are also able to
appreciate or 'perceive' answers. This is another way of saying that
we understand what we are being asked to do and identify the
right answer by using a combination of stored information that is
the result of previous exposure to similar problems. Grasshoppers
are 'recognising' the answer because they identify (albeit without
thinking consciously about it) a calculation they have experienced
before.

This book is written both for inchworms and grasshoppers; it
provides an explanation of number systems and formulae for the
inchworm to use and for the grasshopper to validate their answers.
Whether you feel you are an inchworm or a grasshopper, an
overview of these number systems and formulae is provided in order
to increase your confidence.

However, we need to take care when presented with numbers, as
there are lots of examples within our working environment where
numbers are presented to us in a particular way to have maximum
visual impact in order to make a point. Offering numbers so that we
visualise them in a particular way can lead us to certain conclusions.

We use many examples of charts in care environments. If you
look at the temperature chart (Figure 4.1) you will see that it is
designed in such a way that we can assimilate information easily
and quickly. The solid line running across the chart in the section
indicating temperature represents the 'normal' temperature. This
enables us to see that this patient's temperature has been relatively
stable, but there have been two episodes of a raised temperature.

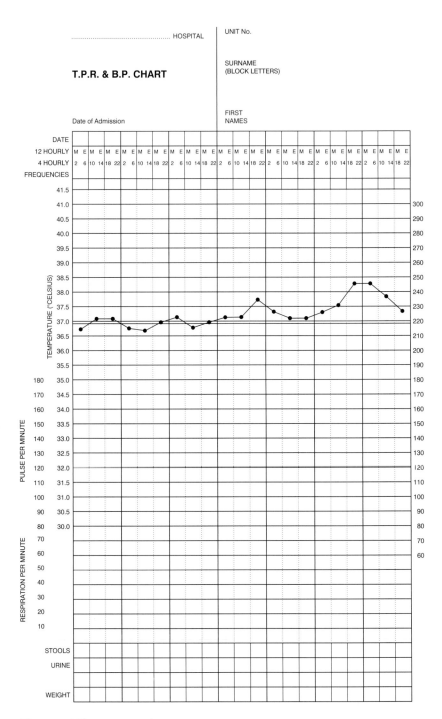

Figure 4.1 *Temperature chart*

However, bar charts and graphs can also be used to persuade us that things are better or worse that we imagine them to be, e.g. profits for a retail company or statistics relating to wound infections.

How we present numbers can be very persuasive. For example, if you were the managing director of a cosmetic company wanting to sell a newly developed 'stay young forever' cream, tested on a small sample, would you want to say that out of 10 women who tested the cream, seven noticed a difference in their skin texture? Or would you rather promote your product by saying that 70% of women noticed a difference? If you used the percentage you would be telling the truth, as seven out of 10 women can be expressed as 70% – but the size of the group interviewed can be very important, for example when trying to determine the validity of some research.

There are important clinical examples where number recognition is vital. When considering whether a patient is overweight, it is important to consult a BMI chart which compares weight with height (see Figure 4.2).

Another important example that arises in children's nursing is the use of percentile charts. These are very similar to the chart above, but compare age and weight.

On a more daily basis we use blood pressure and pulse charts to record observations, and important clinical decisions are made as a consequence of these measurements. It is important to remember that the decisions are based on trends. While a blood pressure measurement that is higher than the normal range for a specific patient is always considered seriously, the measurement is repeated before any action is taken, to see if there is a trend. An observation chart is therefore a common example of a graph used regularly in practice.

Nursing calculations

Over to you

Try to identify four or five different types of calculation that you would use in nursing practice.

Much of the literature (Lapham and Agar 2003; Wright 2005) identifies calculations related to medicine doses, whether oral or intravenous, so you could count these as two examples of calculations. You could probably easily identify dietary/nutritional

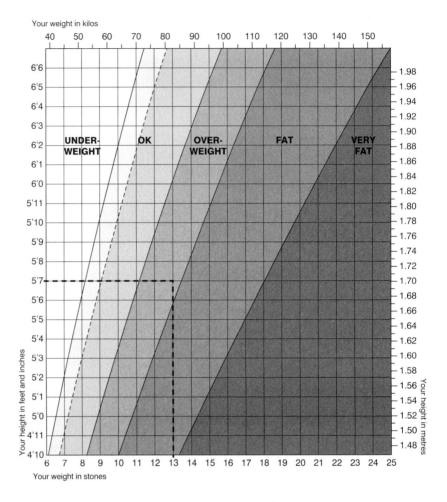

Figure 4.2 *Are you the right weight for your height?*
Source: Food Standards Agency (2006) www.eatwell.gov.uk/healthydiet/
healthyweight/heightweightchart/

needs such as calories or grams of fat, and perhaps even research/
audit calculations, but then you might struggle.

Other examples would be when measuring fluid balance, when
using risk assessment tools such as those used to predict pressure
area damage, or when making sense of statistical information
presented within research articles to promote a particular approach
to care.

This book will take you through many of these and others, but
first you need to consider how accurate we need to be in these
different scenarios.

Rounding up numbers

In the queue for the supermarket checkout you probably round up numbers, so, for example, you expect the shopping bill to be about £15, and therefore expect approximately £5 change from your £20 note. In this situation this is all you need. We tend to automatically round our approximations up to twos, fives and tens, as these are easy numbers to work with and will give us a reasonable approximation.

Even if we wish to make a more accurate guess, we often round up to the nearest five or ten and then subtract the difference. Buying a large container for the garden for £37, plants worth £26, and compost for £9, it is easier to round up to £40 + £30 + £10 (giving an answer of £80) and subtract the difference between the original numbers and the 'tens', £3 + £4 + £1 (£8). The sum then becomes £80 – £8 = £72.

These are strategies we employ for making the numbers, and therefore the calculation, more manageable and easy to calculate in our heads. If we employ strategies such as these, we have a way of confirming our answers are correct as we have an esitmate by which we can judge them.

Rounding up numbers in clinical areas needs special thought. Consider the example of intravenous fluid replacement. We may calculate that the patient requires the fluid to be infused at 41·2 drops per minute. While the amount of fluid to be replaced is important for patients as over-transfusion for example, particularly for the young and old, can be catastrophic, you cannot measure a part of a drop. What we would do in this situation is to round up to the nearest whole number, in this case 42 drops. (There is an argument for rounding figures to the nearest whole number, for example 41·1 to 41·49 round down to 41, and 41·5 to 41·9 round up to 42, but it has become 'custom and practice' to always round up to the next whole number for intravenous fluid drip rates.)

When measuring body fluids such as vomit, urine or wound drainage, we can only measure amounts based upon the equipment we have available, and the measuring jug may measure in amounts of 5 ml. This might be acceptable, but in some cases, for example measurement of medicine dosages and **raytec gauze** counts, precision is critical (Woodrow 1998). Therefore, you should know which calculations in your clinical area need to be exact, and where approximations can be used.

○━▄ *Keywords*

Raytec gauze
The gauze used during surgery. It contains a radio opaque strip so that it can be detected by x-ray

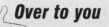

> ## Over to you
>
> Use your Trust's policy to identify when calculations need to be exact.

However, it is always useful to have a rough estimate, as with the grocery shopping, so that you can identify whether your answer is a reasonable one.

Student nurses attending workshops for medicine calculations were asked to work through a sheet of calculations related to medicine doses and have their answers checked as they completed each one. Having reached an answer, students were asked if they thought their answer was a reasonable one, and then sent to test the calculation, i.e. measure the liquid, dispense the tablets, set the intravenous drip rate, etc.

One question set related to a dose of aspirin. One student was very sure that the correct answer was ¼ tablet. She was asked to dispense this dose. After several minutes she came back and stated that she could not do this, although she had tried some very innovative strategies such as diluting a soluble aspirin (which was not on her prescription sheet) and dividing the volume by four. The correct answer was four tablets, and she could have saved herself some time (and resources) if she had an approximate answer to compare with.

In clinical areas, the more practice we have in undertaking calculation, the more skilled we become at estimating. Hutton (1998, p. 38) describes this as 'developing a common sense knowledge of what is a reasonable answer for a particular patient'.

Estimating

If you carry out a calculation and are unsure about your answer, even though you have checked your calculation and used the correct formula/strategy, you can probably confirm your answer in a different way. For example, Woodrow (1998) suggests that the medication dose obtained can be compared with the normal dose ranges within the British National Formulary (BNF).

Preston (2004) suggests that there are checks within the calculation process that nurses can use to make sure the answer they obtain is a reasonable one. For example, if a stock medicine is available in syrup containing 60 mg in 10 ml, and the patient requires 45 mg, we can ask ourselves whether the answer is likely to be less or more than 10 ml.

Whole numbers

Let us start by reminding ourselves of the properties of whole numbers. All whole numbers have only noughts following the decimal point. We tend not to write the noughts as they have no importance unless we are involved in calculation.

For example, if we want to halve 1, it will give us a smaller number than 1 and so we will need to use the decimal point. This is a very straightforward example – we know without thinking about it that half of 1 is a half. We can write our answer in words, but there are other ways of writing this answer. If we were to carry out the calculation on paper as a division, it would look like this:

$$2\overline{)\,1}$$

but we would need to put in the decimal point and a nought in order for it to be clear, thus:

$$2\overline{)1.0}$$

We can then carry out the division: 2 into 1 does not go so, we move the decimal point (one place to the right) to get the number 10 which 2 goes into 5 times. However, the answer then needs to reflect the decimal point so we move the decimal point back (one place to the left), making 5 into 0.5 thus:

$$\frac{0.5}{2\overline{)1.0}}$$

This answer is expressed as a *decimal fraction*.

We could have carried out the calculation in a different way, expressing the calculation as:

$$1 \div 2$$

which could be written as ½.

In this example we need to remember that when whole numbers are expressed as fractions (as the half ½) they are always placed over 1, thus 1 becomes ¹/₁. The division 1 ÷ 2 can then be written as:

$$\frac{1}{1} \div \frac{2}{1}$$

When we divide fractions, we turn the second fraction upside down and multiply:

$$\frac{1}{1} \div \frac{2}{1} = \frac{1}{1} \times \frac{1}{2} = \frac{1}{2}$$

We now have three different expressions for the same amount/value: in words (half), as a decimal (0·5) and as a fraction (¹/₂).

In a calculation you need to choose the most appropriate way of expression, e.g. for a liquid where the calculation is expressed in millilitres, 0·5 ml is a measurable amount using a syringe or calibrated medicine pot whereas ¹/₂ ml is not.

Juxtaposition

Sometimes we get the calculation wrong because we do not understand what we are being asked to do. Consider the following examples.

a. A patient is prescribed an injection of 25 mg of medicine X. The ampoule contains 40 mg per 5 ml. What volume would you draw up into the syringe?

b. Ward stock ampoules contain medicine X in a concentration of 40 mg per 5 ml. Calculate the volume required to give the patient a dose of 25 mg.

c. A patient is prescribed an injection of 40 mg. The ampoule contains 25 mg per 5 ml. What volume does the patient require?

Pause for a moment to consider what you are being asked to do in each of these examples. Examples a and b are actually asking you the same question but in a different way – the information is presented in a different order. Although example c uses the same numbers, it is asking a different question. Sometimes, because of the way we perceive the numbers, we can undertake a calculation the wrong way. The way the information is combined or arranged (juxtaposed) means that it can be misinterpreted, so we need to make sure we understand what we are being asked to do. Cartwright (1996) suggests that students have difficulty with this type of question because of the need to distinguish the dose from the stock strength.

Wright (2005) undertook action research into the most effective way of teaching medicine calculations. She observed that one repeated problem was that when students were asked to find the fraction $^2/_3$, instead of dividing the top number (called the **numerator**) by the bottom number (called the **denominator**), i.e. dividing the 2 by the 3, they actually divided 3 by 2.

If you are getting some calculations wrong, it may be because you do not understand what you are being asked to do. This might be because you have problems with the skills of addition, subtraction, multiplication and division (the *rules of arithmetic* or *number operations*), you do not understand the order in which you need to carry out these calculations (BODMAS) or you cannot interpret the written element of the question. Hutton (1998, p. 2) supports this view. She suggests that when numeracy problems are 'written in words' this adds to their difficulty.

One problem in understanding what we are being asked to do relates to the language used in the instructions we are given. For example, if we are asked to add numbers together, terms used could be 'add', 'plus', 'sum' and 'total'.

Keywords

Numerator
Mathematical jargon for the word used in division to describe the number above the line in a fraction

Denominator
Mathematical jargon for the word used in division to describe the number below the line in a fraction

Over to you

Identify two terms that might be used for each of the following:

1. Subtraction
2. Multiplication
3. Division.

(Answers to this *Over to you* exercise can be found in Appendix D.)

We not only need to understand what we are being asked to do, but we need to know *how* to do it (planning).

BODMAS

When these rules of number/number operations are used within one complex calculation, it is important to do them in the right order (Kearsley Bullen 2003), thus:

B   brackets
pO   powers/roots
D   division

M   multiplication
A   addition
S   subtraction

Let us look at the example.

$12 - 3 \times 2$

Using the BODMAS order, multiplication is carried out before subtraction, so we would multiply the 3×2 first (6) and then subtract it from 12, giving us the answer 6, i.e.

$12 - (3 \times 2) = 12 - 6 = 6$

If we were to ignore BODMAS then we might calculate this as:

$(12 - 3) \times 2$

which translates into $9 \times 2 = 18$.

Over to you

Refresher – using BODMAS

a. $31 - 7 \times 4 =$

b. $28 \times 8 - 17 =$

c. $14 \div 2 \times 7 =$

d. $24 + 49 \div 7 - 18 =$

Number systems

Fractions

Vulgar fractions

We have already identified fractions (also referred to as vulgar fractions). This is where the value of a number is expressed by placing the number *over* a number, e.g. on p. 59 we saw that the whole number 1 written as a fraction would be written as $^1/_1$. One quarter (part of a whole number) becomes $^1/_4$. This is described as a proper fraction because the number on the bottom is the larger number.

The whole number of eight, written as a fraction, becomes $8/1$. This is described as an improper fraction because the number on top is the larger number. We can easily convert this back to a whole number by dividing the numerator 8 by the denominator 1.

Let's examine the fraction $21/6$. This is 21 sixths. There are 6 sixths in every whole, just as there are 8 eighths in every whole, or 9 ninths, etc.

We can see that if we divide the denominator 6 into the numerator 21, it would give us a whole number, but not exactly.

The answer would be $3\tfrac{3}{6}$ because 6 goes into 21 three whole times (which gives us 18) but then we have 3 left over to make 21, making three parts of a sixth or $3/6$.

We could simplify this and write it as $3\tfrac{1}{2}$. We look at simplifying fractions next.

Simplifying fractions

We do this by identifying common factors of the numerator and denominator (numbers that will divide into both).

For example, $12/18$ simplifies into $2/3$ by dividing both the 12 and 18 in the original fraction by 6 (which is a common factor of 12 and 18 as both can be divided equally by 6 to leave a whole number each; put another way, both 12 and 18 are multiples of 6 and this makes 6 a common factor).

However, these are straightforward numbers. Sometimes we start dividing both numbers with, for example, a 2 (only for even numbers) or a 5 (if the numbers end in a 5 or 0) and we might have to do this several times in order to simplify. Obviously this will work with other small numbers such as 3s, 4s, etc.

NB: When we are working with denominators of 10, 100 or 1,000, we tend to leave these as they are easier numbers to work with than their simpler counterparts, e.g. 25, 50. For example, $16/100$ is usually easier to work with than $4/25$.

Adding or subtracting fractions

Consider the following calculation, where we have added fractions:

$$\frac{3}{10} + \frac{5}{10} = \frac{8}{10}$$

All we had to do with this example is add the numbers on the top of the line (*numerators*) because the number below the line (*denominator*) in both fractions is the same.

A useful way of helping you to envisage this is by offering a visual representation, for example:

³/10

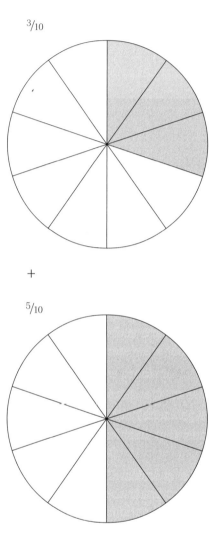

+

⁵/10

If we add the shaded sections together we get 8, but we need to remember to put the 8 over 10 thus ⁸/10, because, as we can see from the pie charts, the shaded sections are part of the whole number of sections, in this case 10.

We can then simplify this number to ⁴/5 by dividing with the same number (in this case 2, because it divides equally into the numerator and denominator). But as we identified above, when the bottom number is 10 it is easier to manage if we leave it as it is.

This example works because the denominators, in this case 10, are the same in both fractions. It would not work where the denominator is different, so we need to find a different approach.

Look at the following example:

$$\frac{8}{10} + \frac{12}{24}$$

We are trying to add two different quantities, so we need to make both quantities the same.

Again you might understand this more easily if you envisage it thus:

$^8/_{10}$

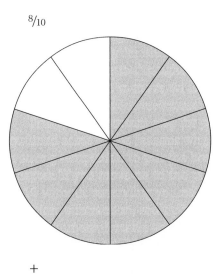

+

$^{12}/_{24}$

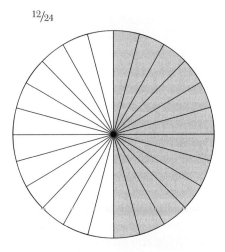

One way to manage this would be to multiply the two denominators, the 10 and 24, so that each fraction has a *new* denominator of 240.

However, whatever we do to the denominator we would have to do to the numerator, so if we multiply 10 (the number on the bottom) by 24, we also need to multiply the 8 (the number on the top) by 24, so we now have $^{192}/_{240}$.

Likewise for the second fraction, we multiplied the number on the bottom by 10, so we need to do the same to the 12, which is $^{120}/_{240}$.

We can now add these together and simplify the answer if we wish.

$$\frac{192 + 120}{240} = \frac{312}{240} = \frac{156}{120} = \frac{13}{10} = 1\frac{3}{10}$$

The first answer involved big numbers and so we simplified this by dividing the numbers above and below the line by 12, but you might find it easier if you use a series of simplifications, e.g. 2 as both numbers are even numbers. Because the numerators were bigger numbers than the denominators, it means that we have some whole numbers in the answer and should reflect this, hence the final answer.

Subtraction of fractions uses the same principles

$$\frac{12}{24} - \frac{8}{24} = \frac{4}{24}$$

We could simplify by dividing both numbers in the answer by 4, thus $^1/_6$.

However, try to subtract different numbers such as

$$\frac{7}{8} - \frac{8}{10}$$

We are trying to subtract different quantities and so we need to convert this into the same quantities by applying the same rule as in addition, e.g.:

$$\frac{70}{80} - \frac{48}{80} = \frac{22}{80} = \frac{11}{40}$$

That is, multiplying the two bottom numbers ($8 \times 10 = 80$), and then simplifying the answer.

Or we could find a number that both the 8 and the 10 divide into, in this case 40, and so the subtraction would now look like this:

$$\frac{7 \times 5}{8 \times 5} - \frac{6 \times 4}{10 \times 4} = \frac{35 - 24}{40} = \frac{11}{40}$$

> ## Over to you
>
> ### Refresher – adding and simplifying fractions
> Check your understanding by adding, subtracting and, where appropriate, simplifying the following fractions
>
> a. $\quad \dfrac{7}{8} + \dfrac{5}{8} + \dfrac{1}{8} =$
>
> b. $\quad \dfrac{3}{11} + \dfrac{6}{11} + \dfrac{1}{11} =$
>
> c. $\quad \dfrac{5}{9} + \dfrac{1}{3} + \dfrac{4}{9} =$
>
> d. $\quad \dfrac{4}{21} + \dfrac{8}{21} + \dfrac{3}{7} =$
>
> e. $\quad \dfrac{5}{6} - \dfrac{3}{6} =$
>
> f. $\quad \dfrac{5}{18} - \dfrac{2}{9} =$
>
> g. $\quad \dfrac{5}{6} - \dfrac{4}{9} =$
>
> h. $\quad \dfrac{7}{16} + \dfrac{4}{16} - \dfrac{5}{8} =$

Multiplying and dividing fractions

When we multiply fractions we can simply multiply the numerators and denominators.

$$\frac{15}{18} \times \frac{12}{9} = \frac{15 \times 12}{18 \times 9} = \frac{180}{162}$$

or

$$\frac{\cancel{15}^{5}}{\cancel{18}^{6}} \times \frac{\cancel{12}^{4}}{\cancel{9}^{3}} = \frac{5 \times 4}{6 \times 3} = \frac{20}{18}$$

Here, 3 is a common factor of 15 and 18, and also for the 12 and 9. If we simplify the answer of $^{20}/_{18}$ we have $^{10}/_{9}$ which can be further simplified to $1^{1}/_{9}$.

> ### Over to you
>
> **Refresher – multiplying and simplifying fractions**
>
> Check your understanding by adding, subtracting and where appropriate simplifying fractions
>
> a. $\dfrac{4}{7} \times \dfrac{5}{8} =$
>
> b. $\dfrac{3}{12} \times \dfrac{8}{14} =$
>
> c. $\dfrac{5}{9} \times \dfrac{8}{9} =$
>
> d. $\dfrac{7}{11} \times \dfrac{4}{5} =$

Dividing fractions is a very simple process, as we just turn the second fraction upside down, simplify the fractions and multiply the numerators and denominators:

$$\frac{15}{18} \div \frac{12}{9} \quad \text{becomes} \quad \frac{15}{18} \times \frac{9}{12}$$

$$\frac{\cancel{15}^{5}}{\cancel{18}^{2}} \times \frac{\cancel{9}^{1}}{\cancel{12}^{4}} = \frac{5}{2} \times \frac{1}{4} = \frac{5}{8}$$

> ### Over to you
>
> **Refresher – dividing and simplifying fractions**
>
> a. $\dfrac{1}{3} \div \dfrac{1}{5} =$
>
> b. $\dfrac{3}{7} \div \dfrac{3}{5} =$
>
> d. $\dfrac{9}{17} \div \dfrac{10}{11} =$
>
> d. $\dfrac{17}{21} \div \dfrac{9}{11} =$

As we established above, any vulgar fraction can be written as a decimal fraction by dividing the denominator into the numerator. So $^5/_8$ can be expressed as $0\cdot625$ because 5 divided by 8 = 0.625.

We call this a decimal fraction. To change this back to a vulgar fraction we put the decimal fraction over 1,000. The number of noughts is determined by how many numbers there are after the decimal point. In 0.625 there are three numbers so we need to move the decimal point three places to the right, to make 625 over 1,000 (with three noughts). This means that the decimal point is no longer needed. This results in somewhat unwieldy numbers and so using common factors (25 and then 5) we can simplify this.

$$\frac{625}{1,000} = \frac{625^{25}}{1,000^{40}} = \frac{25^5}{40^8} = \frac{5}{8}$$

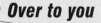

Over to you

Refresher – changing vulgar fractions to decimal fractions

Change the following to decimal fractions

a. $\frac{2}{7}$ =

b. $\frac{5}{4}$ =

c. $\frac{8}{11}$ =

d. $\frac{7}{8}$ =

The decimal system

It is important to remember that a whole number, such as 1, has *trailing* zeros which we would not normally write, but we could put any amount of trailing zeros *after* the decimal point in a whole number, e.g. 1·0, 1·00 or 1·000. Whole numbers also have *leading* zeros that are not usually written because like the trailing zero they make no difference to the value, e.g. 01, 001, and 0001. However, zeros become very important when they are in the middle of numbers, e.g. 101, or if they are *before* a decimal point, e.g. 0·1, as they indicate the value of the number (Kearsley Bullen 2003). For example, 2·0 indicates the number 2, whereas 0·2 represents an amount ten times smaller (because the decimal point is one place further to the right). Kapborg (1995) reports that putting the decimal point in the wrong place is a common error that student nurses make when calculating.

Table 4.1 Place value

Thousands	Hundreds	Tens	Ones	Decimal point	Tenths	Hundredths
8	0	7	5	.	1	0

Sometimes it makes it easier if we visualise this system as a diagram showing the 'tens'; this helps locate numbers in appropriate columns. If we take the example of eight thousand and seventy-five point one, this would be expressed in numbers as 8075·1.

Table 4.1 is an example of how to express numbers using the decimal system. Each column represents a number ten times smaller or larger than the number next to it (Kearsley Bullen 2003). It helps us recap on some points we introduced above when we were discussing the properties of numbers.

We can distinguish large numbers by the use of commas, i.e. there can be a comma after the thousand. There are any amount of noughts after the decimal point that we do not usually identify, but we always identify *numbers* after the decimal point. Just to clarify this, 0·1 could be written as 0·1000, but there would be no purpose to this. However, noughts in the middle of a number 0·102, are always written.

Place value

Decimal points are so easily misread that they should be avoided in clinical practice wherever possible (Gregory 2002; BNF 2006). However, this is not always possible and some medication given to children and older people is prescribed in small doses. Pharmacies will try to minimise the risk of error by providing the medication in a smaller unit, so you need to understand SI units and also be able to multiply and divide using decimal fractions. SI units are considered in Chapter 5.

We know that when using decimal fractions, whole numbers have a trailing zero (Hutton 2003) which is not usually written. For example, the whole number 1, if written with its trailing zero, would be expressed as 1·0. The reason we leave off the zero is that it could be easily mistaken for 10, but we do use the zeros during calculations. On the other hand, leading zeros are always used. When expressing decimals that have a value of less than 1, we should always precede it with a nought, e.g. 0·1, which if written without the zero, as ·1, could be mistaken for 1 (Hutton 2003).

We use conventions of commas and full stops to indicate the size of numbers. The previous examples used a full stop to indicate a decimal point, but if written in words the examples would be 'one point nought' and 'nought point one' respectively. Commas are used in numbers over a thousand, thus: 1,000 to indicate one thousand, and 10,000 to indicate ten thousand (Hutton 2003).

When undertaking a calculation you may be asked to state a value to a number of decimal places. This refers to the number of figures after the decimal point. Thus 4·77 is stated to two decimal places, whereas 4·7 is stated to one decimal place.

Consider the following:

12,345 indicates twelve thousand, three hundred and forty-five

1,234·5 indicates one thousand, two hundred and thirty-four point five

0·12345 indicates zero point one two three four five.

So we can conclude that moving the digits of a number one place to the left makes it bigger (by a factor of 10) and moving the digits one place to the right makes it smaller (by a factor of 10).

It is easier if we express this in numbers:

> 1·2345
> 12·345
> 123·45
> 1234·5

and

> 12·345
> 1·2345
> 0·12345
> 0·012345

✍ *Over to you*

Refresher – decimals

a. Write 444·44 in words

b. Express two thousand, two hundred and twenty in figures

c. Multiply 4·4 by 1,000

d. Divide 222·2 by 10.

Change the following to vulgar fractions, and simplify where possible:

a. 0·55 =

b. 0·72 =

c. 0·68 =

d. 0·09 =

Moving on – application to practice

According to Haigh (2002) and Blais and Bath (1992), nurses find most difficulty with calculations that involve ratios, percentages, fractions and place value. Having looked at fractions and place value, we will now take you through ratios and percentages.

Ratios

Ratios enable you to compare numbers or amounts. So if in a fully occupied ward of 30 beds designated as surgical beds, five contain patients who have been moved from the medical ward, then the ratio of medical to surgical patients would be 5:25. In other words, while five of the beds contain patients who have a medical condition, the remaining beds (30 – 5) contain patients with surgical conditions.

We can simplify this ratio, as both 5 and 25 are divisible by 5. If we divide both numbers in the ratio by 5 we would report a ratio of 1:5 medical to surgical patients. Take another example where there are seven empty beds in a ward of 30 beds. This would give us the ratio 7:23 of empty to occupied beds. This ratio does not simplify easily (dividing by 7 gives 1:3·29, but this could be rounded down to approximately 1:3).

Ratios are often used when expressing strengths, for example the strength of the medication adrenaline, which can be expressed as 1:1,000 or 1:10,000. Numbers are meaningless unless we can assign some context to them, in this case 1 gram of adrenalin to 1,000 or 10,000 millilitres of fluid. Grams and millilitres are units of measurement used in the SI system.

If there are seven qualified nurses on duty, but the total number of nursing staff is 12, then the number of unqualified staff would be the difference between the total number (12) and the number of qualified nurses (7), i.e. five unqualified staff. The ratio of qualified to unqualified staff would be 7:5. It is easy to confuse this and assume the ratio is 7:12.

⤳ *Over to you*

Refresher – ratios

Calculate the following ratios:

a. Four patients in the ward of 30 are ready for discharge – what is the ratio of patients ready for discharge to patients remaining?

b. Eight out of 24 beds are occupied – what is the ratio of occupied to empty beds?

c. There are six empty beds in a ward of 24 beds – what is the ratio of empty to occupied beds?

d. Of the 24 patients in the ward, three have the blood group AB – what is the ratio of patients with blood group AB to patients with another blood group?

Percentages

Percentages are usually used to indicate 'parts per hundred' (Hutton 2003).

If we take the example above of bed occupancy, but wish to express this as a percentage rather than ratio, for example the percentage of bed occupancy during one week in May, we would use the following formula:

$$\text{percentage value} = \frac{\text{value of item being measured} \times 100}{\text{total number of items in system}}$$

(James *et al.* 2002)

Suppose during our identified week, 24 out of 36 beds were continuously occupied, then this would be expressed as a percentage in the following way:

$$\text{percentage value} = \frac{24 \times 100}{36}$$

This would reflect a percentage of 66·6 (recurring). 'Recurring' means that we can write any amount of the figure 6 after the decimal point. If we want to state the answer to one decimal place, we round it up to 66·7.

If we read that within a school 6% of the children have green eyes, this means that of every 100 children in the school, six children have green eyes.

Many lotions, ointments, medicines and intravenous fluids are available in different strengths. A very straightforward example of this is Daktarin, a cream available over the counter for the treatment of athlete's foot. The label states that there is 20 mg miconazole per gram, which is 2%. This is explained below.

So per cent refers to parts per hundred or hundredths. If we take the example of 5% of 20, this can be written in several different ways, but they will only be meaningful if we remember that the 'of' refers to 'multiplied by'. Thus:

$$5\% \text{ (5 hundredths)} = \frac{5}{100}$$

To find 5% of 20 we now multiply this fraction by 20:

$$\frac{5}{100} \times 20 = \frac{\cancel{100}}{\cancel{100}} = \frac{1}{1}$$

If we cancel out the noughts we are left with $^1/_1$.

With vulgar fractions like this we divide the bottom into the top to get 1.

But as we know, whole numbers as vulgar fractions are expressed as the whole number over 1, which leaves us again with the number 1.

These were easy numbers to work with. Suppose we wanted to express 6% of 41. We would go through the same process:

$$6\% \text{ (6 hundredths)} = \frac{6}{100}$$

Then multiply this by 41:

$$\frac{6}{100} \times 41 = \frac{246}{100} = 2\frac{46}{100} = 2.46$$

As a decimal fraction this would be 2.46.

In the previous example of Daktarin cream, in order to calculate the percentage of miconazole in this ointment we need to turn the **equation** upside down, thus:

$$\frac{20 \text{ mg}}{1 \text{ g}}$$

However, we need to make sure both SI units are the same. As the gram is the bigger unit, if we convert this to milligrams, the smaller unit, we would need to express 1 gram as 1,000 milligrams. Our calculation now looks like this:

$$\frac{20}{1,000} \times 100 = \frac{2,000}{100} = \frac{2}{1} = 2$$

Thus we see that there is 2% miconazole in Daktarin.

⊙━ Keywords

Equation
Mathematical shorthand which expresses the calculation to be carried out. One side of the equals sign is equivalent to the other side

In health care we use percentages in a range of situations, for example patients returning from theatre with intravenous therapy in situ could be receiving an infusion of 5% glucose.

Over to you

Refresher – percentages

Calculate the following percentages:

a. Six empty beds in a ward of 24 beds
b. Eighteen occupied beds in a ward of 24 beds
c. What percentage is 120 g of 200 g?
d. What percentage is 12 g of 150 g?

Formulae

There are two sets of formulae/processes which can be helpful when determining doses for medicines: one for oral medication and one for intravenous medication.

Working out the correct dose of an oral medication

Standard dose requirements

You may need to calculate the number of tablets, volume for injection, or volume of medicine required.

The formula we use for this is:

$$\text{dose} = \frac{\text{strength required} \times \text{stock volume}}{\text{strength available}}$$

or

$$\text{what we need} = \frac{\text{what we want} \times \text{the amount it comes in}}{\text{what we have}}$$

For example:

James is prescribed 300 mg of aspirin, the stock available is 75 mg per tablet.

$$\text{dose needed} = \frac{300 \times 1}{75} = \frac{300}{75} = 4 \text{ tablets}$$

We can also apply this formula to injections.

For example:

Rashid is prescribed 0·3 mg of medicine Y. The stock ampoule contains 0·4 mg per ml. How much of the drug would you need to draw up into the syringe?

$$\text{dose needed} = \frac{0.3}{0.4} \times 1 \text{ ml}$$

We may wish to get rid of the decimal point by multiplying both doses by 10. NB: The answer will not need to be changed, as we have made the same alteration to the numbers on top and below the line.

$$\frac{3 \times 1}{4} = \frac{3}{4} \text{ ml}$$

We now need to convert this to a decimal fraction to draw up the required volume, i.e. 0·75 ml.

Over to you

Refresher – calculating oral medicines

You have a medicine dispensed as 400 milligrams in 20 millilitres. How many millilitres will you give if the doctor orders:

a. 80 milligrams?

b. 120 milligrams?

c. 50 milligrams?

d. 60 milligrams?

Using medicines expressed as percentages

Suppose the prescription for Mrs Gera asks you to administer 50 mg Lidocaine, using an ampoule containing Lidocaine expressed as a percentage, in this case 1%.

To determine the amount to administer, we need to go through the following steps.

If the ampoule contains 100 ml fluid, a percentage of 1% means that there is 1 gram of the Lidocaine per 100 ml fluid. We need to convert the grams to milligrams, as the prescription for the patient is in milligrams. This will tell us how many milligrams of Lidocaine there are in 100 ml fluid.

We could do this in one calculation, as follows.

1%	= 1 gram in 100 ml fluid
1,000 milligrams	= 1 gram
1%	= 1,000 mg in 100 ml fluid

We need to administer 50 mg Lidocaine, so we need to work out how much Lidocaine (mg) is contained in 1 ml of fluid. If there are 1,000 mg per 100 ml, then we can calculate that there will be 10 mg per 1 ml (1,000 ÷ 100).

Dividing by 10 again, we can calculate that there is 1 mg per 0·1 ml, which we need to multiply by 50 to find the volume of fluid (ml) we need to draw up into the syringe.

volume to be drawn up =

$$\frac{50 \text{ (mg dose required)} \times 100 \text{ (ml per ampoule)}}{1,000 \text{ (mg per ampoule)}} =$$

5 ml (of Lidocaine)

Weight-related doses

If you are required to work out the single dose of a medicine related to a patient's body weight, the formula would look like this:

single dose =

$$\frac{\text{recommended dose (per kilogram)} \times \text{body weight (kilograms)}}{\text{number of doses per day}}$$

Mrs Zimmerman is prescribed 5 mg of Gentamycin per kilogram of her body weight. This is to be divided into four equal doses. She weighs 78 kilograms.

single dose =

$$\frac{\text{recommended dose (5 mg/kg)} \times \text{body weight (78 kg)}}{\text{number of doses per day (4)}}$$

$$= \frac{5 \times 78}{4} = \frac{390}{4} = 97.5 \text{ mg}$$

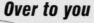

Over to you

Refresher – weight related doses

A patient is to receive a dose of 5 mg per kg of body weight, per day, divided into four equal doses. What would be the individual dose for the following?

a. The patient weighs 64 kg

b. The patient weighs 72 kg

c. The patient weighs 76 kg

d. The patient weighs 80 kg

Intravenous infusion rates

To work out an intravenous infusion rate using a manually controlled infusion system, we use the following formula:

$$\text{rate} = \frac{\text{volume}}{\text{time}}$$

Consider the following prescription: Mr Judge is to receive 1 litre of 0.9% sodium chloride over a period of six hours.

If we use the formula above we will find that it has some limitations.

$$\text{rate} = \frac{\text{volume (one litre} = 1,000 \text{ ml)}}{\text{time (6 hours)}}$$

$$\text{rate} = \frac{1,000 \text{ ml/h}}{6 \text{ hours}}$$

This calculation will provide us with an answer, but it will be stated as ml per hour. We need to be able to count drops, either by using a watch or a drop counter, and so we need to work out how to establish the number of drops that are contained in a ml. This information is provided on the wrapper of the intravenous infusion administration set. The formula below is a more comprehensive one, which will not only provide us with the number of drops, but also drops per minute, which we would be able to count.

$$\text{rate} = \frac{\text{volume (in ml)} \times \text{drops per ml (drop factor)}}{\text{time (in hours)} \times \text{minutes in an hour}}$$

Suppose we use the prescription for Mr Judge again, and on checking the administration set wrapper we find that there are 20 drops in each ml, then we would establish the answer in drops per minute (dpm).

NB: Most giving sets deliver 20 drops per ml of a clear fluid and 15 drops per ml for blood, but you should always check the information provided by the manufacturer.

rate (drops per minute) =

$$\frac{\text{volume (1,000 ml)} \times \text{drop factor (20)}}{\text{time (6 hours)} \times \text{minutes in an hour (60)}}$$

We can rewrite this thus:

$$\text{rate} = \frac{1,000 \times 20}{6 \times 60}$$

Which would give us an answer of:

$$\frac{20,000}{360} = 55.5 \ldots \text{dpm}$$

We would need to round this up as we cannot count parts of a drop: 56 dpm.

NB: We discussed multiplying fractions and rounding up figures earlier in this chapter.

However, sometimes we use a medical device such as a syringe driver to deliver intravenous fluids. These are based upon the delivery of ml of fluid per hour as are some electronically controlled drop counters.

The formula we use in these cases is simpler, and would look like this:

$$\text{delivery rate (ml per hour)} = \frac{\text{volume (in ml)}}{\text{time (in hours)}}$$

Alternatively, we might come on duty and find that Mr Judge is connected to a syringe driver delivering 100 ml of fluid at 40 ml per hour. He asks you how much longer this infusion will last; you notice there is 80 ml of fluid left in the syringe. We then need to use the following equation:

$$40 \text{ (ml per hour)} = \frac{80 \text{ ml}}{\text{time}}$$

In order to work out this calculation of time we need to turn it around, thus:

$$\text{time} = \frac{80 \text{ ml}}{40 \text{ ml per hour}} = 2 \text{ hours}$$

For a child we may use a different intravenous infusion set, one which incorporates a burette (micro-drop giving set). With children and vulnerable adults such as those in intensive care units we may be concerned about over-transfusion. Having a burette incorporated within the administration set means that we have an extra chamber that will hold a smaller amount of fluid, possibly 100 ml. This effectively means that if the fluid were transfused too quickly then only the fluid in the burette would be transfused, and not the fluid in the 500 ml or 1,000 ml container. The drop rate per ml for this type of delivery is usually 60 drops, so it is important to always check the information on the administration set wrapper provided by the manufacturer.

This information presented in a formula would look like this:

rate (drops per minute) =

$$\frac{\text{volume} \times \text{drop factor (drops per ml) (60)}}{\text{time (in hours)} \times \text{minutes in an hour (60)}}$$

This calculation should be easier because we cancel out the 60 on the top row with the 60 on the bottom row:

rate (drops per minute) =

$$\frac{\text{volume} \times \text{drop factor } (\cancel{60})^{1}}{\text{time (in hours)} \times \text{minutes in an hour } (\cancel{60})^{1}}$$

Suppose that Sunil is to receive 500 ml of 0·9% sodium chloride over a period of eight hours. Using the above formula we would calculate the drip rate thus:

rate (drops per minute) =

$$\frac{\text{volume (500)} \times \text{drop factor } (\cancel{60})^{1}}{\text{time (8)} \times \text{minutes in an hour } (\cancel{60})^{1}}$$

This can be simplified:

$$\text{rate(drops per minute)} = \frac{500 \times 1}{8 \times 1}$$

The rate would then be 62·5 dpm, which would be rounded up to 63 dpm.

Over to you

Refresher – drip rates

Calculate the drip rates for the following:

a. A patient is prescribed 1,000 ml of fluid over eight hours (20 drops per ml)

b. A patient is prescribed 500 ml of fluid over three hours (20 drops per ml)

c. A patient is prescribed 500 ml of fluid over eight hours (60 drops per ml)

d. A patient is prescribed 500 ml of fluid over six hours (60 drops per ml)

You might find these useful; however, you may already use a slightly different technique when calculating. There are different approaches to calculation; the only thing that is important is that you consistently obtain the correct answer.

The other important thing to note about these calculations and formulae is that we have been using ml to describe amounts of fluid, and minutes as units of time. These measurements are examples of SI units. These SI units are identified and explained in Chapter 5.

Conclusions

This chapter has provided an overview of the rules applied to numbers and using numbers, including the formulae used frequently in clinical areas. We have applied these to some clinical examples to make them more meaningful. We have also provided an ongoing dialogue about the issues related to number, such as when accuracy is required. Potential pitfalls have been identified.

> ## ℞℞℞℞℞**Rapid recap**
>
> Check your progress so far by working through each of the following points
> 1. Explain the term 'vulgar fraction'
> 2. How would you convert a vulgar fraction to a decimal fraction?
> 3. Give an example of a formula used to establish the drip rate for an intravenous infusion
> 4. Provide two examples of formulae which could be used for calculating the dose of an oral medication
>
> If you have difficulty with more than one of the questions, read through the section again to refresh your understanding before moving on.

References

Blais, K. and Bath, J. (1992) Drug calculation errors of baccalaureate nursing students. *Nurse Educator*, **17**(1), 12–15.

BMJ Publishing Group and RPS Publishing (2006) *British National Formulary*. www.bnf.org.uk

Carper, B. (1978) Fundamental patterns of knowing in nursing. *Advances in Nursing Science*, **1**, 13–23.

Cartwright, M. (1996) Numeracy needs of the beginning Registered Nurse. *Nurse Education Today*, **16**, 137–143.

Chinn, S. (1998) *Sum Hope. Breaking the Numbers Barrier*. Souvenir Press, London.

Dowding, D. and Thompson, C. (2003) Issues and innovations in nursing practice. *Journal of Advanced Nursing*, **44**(1), 49–59.

Gregory, S. (2002) Writing a prescription. *Practice Nurse*, **25**(4), 24–26.

Haigh, S. (2002) How to calculate drug dose accurately: advice for nurses. *Professional Nurse*, **18**(1), 54–57.

Hutton, B.M. (1998) Nursing mathematics: the importance of application. *Nursing Standard*, **13**(11), 35–38.

Hutton, B.M. (2003) Calculations for new prescribers. *Nursing Standard*, **17**(25), 47–53.

James, J., Baker, C. and Swain, H. (2002) *Principles of Science for Nurses*. Blackwell Science Ltd, Oxford.

Kapborg, I.D. (1994) An evaluation of Swedish nurse students' calculation ability in relation to their earlier educational background. *Nurse Education Today*, **15**(1), 69–74.

Kearsley Bullen, R. (2003) *BBC KS3 Bitesize Revision*. BBC Worldwide, England. See also www.bbc.co.uk/bitesize.

Knight, P. (2001) *Assessment Series No 7 – A Briefing on Key Concepts*. LTSN Generic Centre, York.

Lapham, R. and Agar, H. (2003*) Drug Calculations for Nurses. A Step-by-Step Approach*, 2nd edn. Arnold, London.

Ollerton, M. (2003) *Getting the Buggers to Add Up*. Continuum, London.

Pólya, G. (1990) *How to Solve It: A New Aspect of Mathematical Method*, 2nd edn. Penguin, London.

Preston, R.M. (2004) Drug errors and patient safety: the need for change in practice. *British Journal of Nursing*, **13**(2), 72–79.

Sierpinska, A. (1994) *Understanding in Mathematics*. The Falmer Press, London.

The Times (2005) *Su Doku. The Number-Placing Puzzle*, Book 2. Collins, London.

Woodrow, P. (1998) Numeracy skills. *Nursing Standard*, **12**(30), 48–53.

Wright, K. (2005) An exploration into the most effective way to teach drug calculation skills to student nurses. *Nurse Education Today*, **25**(6), 430–436.

5

An introduction to SI units in health care

Learning outcomes

By the end of this chapter you should be able to:

- Describe the SI units used in health care
- Provide a rationale for the SI units used in health care
- Provide examples from practice of SI units in use

To aid your understanding and use of the formulae that we introduced in Chapter 4, you need to be familiar with the units used for measuring different quantities.

Overview of SI units

In Chapter 3 we used the example of trying to lose weight and identified that some people still think in stones and pounds. We should use the correct measurement, which in this case would be kilograms. The problem with this is that it involves a calculation because we need to convert one to the other, and often need to explain this to patients.

Stones and pounds are an example of an imperial measurement, and in the British health care system there used to be many examples of these – ounces on a fluid balance chart for example (although this actually refers to a fluid ounce). We also used an apothecary system of measurement (for example *grains* of morphine).

Theory to practice

The example of ounces (e.g. flour in a recipe) and fluid ounces is an important one. If we are trying to establish fluid output but are unable to measure fluid, then we can weigh fluid-soaked materials. The underlying principle is that a fluid ounce weighs the same as a dry weight ounce. So if we wanted to establish urinary output for a young baby, we could weigh the nappy. However, it is important to remember that we need to weigh the dry nappy first or we will not get an accurate measurement of the fluid it has absorbed. We now use the SI units for weight and fluid, gram and litre respectively. An example is offered in Chapter 9.

The kilogram is an example of an SI unit (Le Système Internationale d'Unités, i.e. The International System of Units) (Bell 1993). SI units refer to units of measurement, such as mass, length and time. These and other examples are discussed in more detail later in this chapter. The reason for identifying and adopting SI units in Britain was primarily safety. As patients, staff and information travel between countries, it was important to make this as safe as possible. Most of our European colleagues use the metric system. Having to make calculations to convert units introduced a potential for errors to be made. So SI units were introduced into the British health service in 1975 to enhance safe practice and save time.

At that time other measurements, such as the weight of apples in a supermarket or the temperature on a weather chart, were still measured in imperial units, so we used two systems and often converted from one to the other. Since 2000 it has been illegal to sell produce in pounds and ounces. However, there are still some everyday examples of imperial measurements, such as pints of draught beer.

Over to you

Consider examples of measurements you will use on a regular basis and identify two measurements expressed in SI units and two using imperial measurements.

You could have identified weight, pressure, volume, length, temperature and amount of substance as examples of SI units, and speeds and traffic signs as imperial measurements (i.e. a speed limit of 30 'miles' per hour, and roadworks in 200 'yards').

SI units are based on the metric system, which involves using tens, hundreds and thousands. This was felt to be an easier range of numbers to use. However, if we then get this calculation wrong, we can be wrong by tens, hundreds or thousands, which can be disastrous for the patient.

The idea behind SI units is that there is a *base unit* for each of the measurements, i.e. mass or length. We have already mentioned the kilogram. This is the base unit for mass (although we tend to refer to this in clinical settings as weight). If you think about mass/ weight, though, it is possible to be measuring very small amounts such as an ingredient for a recipe, or really large amounts such as the loads transported by haulage firms. It is important to weigh the load accurately in order to assess, for example, whether a lorry is able to cope with the load. A similar example from practice would be assessing the load when moving a patient or transporting boxes containing equipment.

The range of measurements is shown by placing a *prefix* in front of the unit of measurement so we can easily recognise whether we are referring to large or small amounts. Thus, using the prefix 'kilo' in front of 'gram' indicates a heavier load. These prefixes can be used for all units. The prefix always has the same meaning wherever it is used, so adding 'kilo' before the unit will always indicate a large amount (Hutton 2003). In fact kilo refers to a multiple of 1,000. Its symbol 'k' is used in general conversation to indicate this, for example we might discuss a car costing us 7k (£7,000) (www. en.wikipedia.org).

Conventions

Conventions are an emerging set of rules or customs that are applied to situations. There are several conventions applied to SI units. Most prefixes that indicate a bigger unit have the symbol written as a capital letter, those that indicate a smaller unit have the symbol expressed in lower case. There are some exceptions to this, i.e. the prefix 'kilo', as this could be confused with the kelvin, K, the symbol for temperature.

If you consider the information given in Table 5.1, you will see that kilo refers to a thousand. Prefixes added to the units indicate differences in measurements by multiples of ten. This should become clear when you look at the information contained in Table 5.1 (on opposite page).

Hence, we have the term kilogram, millimetre etc. However, only some of these are used on a daily basis in health care. A common example of where these prefixes become important is on medicine doses. One very common example is that of Digoxin (Lanoxin), prescribed for the young or old in a PG (paediatric/geriatric) dose of 0·0625 mg. Because we have numbers after the decimal point, this indicates a small number. Many of us would have difficulty picturing small amounts such as this, and numbers that involve decimal points are felt to be unwieldy and to have potential for errors (Kapborg 1995; Gregory 2002). To minimise this risk, your pharmacy will probably provide the medication in a bottle labelled with the unit micrograms (a smaller unit; the underpinning principle here is that whole numbers are used wherever possible).

This means that you need to be familiar with the information contained in Table 5.1 in order to determine the correct dose. The bottle would be labelled 62·5 micrograms, which is another way of

Table 5.1 Prefixes

Prefix	Symbol	Number (word)	Value
mega-	M	million	1,000,000
kilo-	k***	thousand	1,000
hecto-	h***	hundred	100
deca-*	da***	ten	10
deci-	d	tenth	$^1/10$ (0·1)
centi-	c	hundredth	$^1/100$
milli-	m	thousandth	$^1/1,000$
micro-**	mc	millionth	$^1/1,000,000$
nano-	n	thousand millionth	$^1/1,000,000,000$

*Some texts now refer to this prefix as deka (www.en.wikipedia.org)
**This is often identified as having the greek mu as its symbol. However, in health care this is avoided in order to eliminate error. Check your 'Trust medicine' policy for their stance on this
***These symbols do not follow the rule of using a capital symbol for a bigger unit and a lower case symbol for a smaller unit

stating 0·0625 mg. If we check the table, we can see that there are 1,000 micrograms in a milligram, and to calculate this we need to move the decimal point to the right by three places (because of the three noughts expressed in 1,000), which gives us a bigger number 62·5, but still contains a decimal point.

To be able to work with SI units in this way, we must first be able to recognise the prefixes that denote whether we are using a small or large amount, as denoted by the prefixes identified in Table 5.1. We also need to be able to undertake the conversion to move between the larger and smaller amounts. You may find Table 5.2 useful.

You may find it easier to understand if you see this represented in a diagram (Figure 5.1).

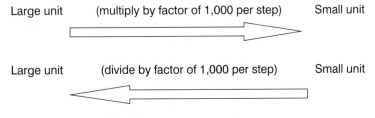

Large unit   (multiply by factor of 1,000 per step)   Small unit

Large unit   (divide by factor of 1,000 per step)   Small unit

Figure 5.1 *Converting units*

Table 5.2 Converting units	
Converting a larger unit to a smaller unit (this involves multiplication)	
Kilogram (kg) to gram (g)	× 1,000
Gram (g) to milligram (mg)	× 1,000
Milligram (mg) to microgram (mcg)	× 1,000
Microgram (mcg) to nanogram (ng)	× 1,000
Converting a smaller unit to a larger unit (this involves division)	
Nanogram (ng) to microgram (mcg)	÷ 1,000
Microgram (mcg) to milligram (mg)	÷ 1,000
Milligram (mg) to gram (g)	÷ 1,000
Gram (g) to kilogram (kg)	÷ 1,000

Whenever we convert a unit in this way, the actual amount remains the same. So although 62·5 looks like a larger amount than 0·0625, we must always consider the SI unit being used – 62·5 micrograms has the same value as 0·0625 milligrams. It is important to remember that the bigger number (62·5) reflects the smaller unit (microgram).

To avoid confusion, 'microgram' is usually written in full. You will need to be familiar with your Trust's Administration of Medicines Policy so that you are sure about their advice on issues such as this.

NB: Although micrograms is plural, the abbreviation is written as mcg and not, as you might expect, as mcgs (Woodrow 1998; Coben and Atere-Roberts 2005). This applies to plurals of all SI units, and the rationale for this is that abbreviations, in whichever clinical context they are used, can be confused.

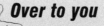

Over to you

Refresher – units of measure

Write the following abbreviations or symbols in full:

a. 1 g =

b. 500 mg =

c. 450 mcg =

d. 2 ml =

How many milligrams in:

a. 1 gram =

b. 0·5 gram =

c. 0·02 gram =

d. 0·005 gram =

Express the following as grams and decimal parts of a gram:

a. 1,500 milligrams =

b. 750 milligrams =

c. 20 milligrams =

d. 1 milligram =

How many micrograms in:

a. 1 milligram =

b. 0·25 milligrams =

c. 0·05 milligrams =

d. 0·001 milligrams =

You have tablets strength 150 milligrams each. How many tablets will you give if the doctor orders:

a. 0·3 gram =

b. 0·45 gram =

c. 0·6 gram =

d. 0·15 gram =

You have tablets strength 10 milligrams each. How many tablets will you give if the doctor orders:

a. 0·05 gram =

b. 0·02 gram =

c. 0·1 gram =

d. 0·01 gram =

In nursing practice we sometimes forget to use the SI unit. Think about the advice we are given to reduce our cholesterol levels. At the time of writing, the advice is to maintain a level of 4 or below. But 4 what? If you visit the website www.lesscholesterol.co.uk you will find that the level refers to 4 mmol/litre. The lack of a unit can be very confusing for patients as well as staff. There is a very common example of where we do this in clinical practice. If you consult a fluid balance chart you will probably find that drinks and urinary output are recorded as numbers only – for example, 180. There might be a reference to the SI units, in this case millilitres, at the bottom of the chart.

Also, consider how we express blood-pressure measurements. For example, we often talk about a patient's blood pressure as being 120 over 70 (120/70). This actually refers to 120/70 mm Hg (Hg being the chemical symbol for mercury). We used to measure blood pressure using equipment that involved reading a column of mercury, and it was easier to envisage how the numbers related to the height of the column of mercury when listening to where the Korotkoff sounds appear and disappear.

SI units

To recap, a unit is a specific measure for a physical quantity such as length. These are further described as *base* units and *derived* units. A base unit reflects a single measurement such as length, whereas a derived unit is one that is formed by combining a number of base units which amalgamates the different measurements. Examples of derived units used in health care are concentration, volume and density.

Base units

There are seven base units (Bell 1993), but in health care we use the base units for: length, mass, amount of substance and temperature.

You are probably familiar with the units identified in Table 5.3. The table shows the SI unit, what it measures and its symbol (how we indicate the SI unit).

We will now discuss in more detail the significance of these for health care.

Length

If we were asked to give an example of length we could easily identify the length of a ruler or a football pitch. However, length

Table 5.3 Base units

Quantity	SI unit	Symbol
Length	metre	m
Mass	kilogram	kg
Amount of substance	mole	mol
Temperature	kelvin	K

is a common measurement in health care. For example, since the concern about methicillin resistant *Staphyloccus aureus* (MRSA) there are guidelines about distances between beds and sinks (NHS Estates 2003).

We measure length in many different clinical contexts. For example, to establish whether a patient is overweight we need to know the patient's height. We use different lengths of needle when carrying out an injection, depending upon which tissue we need to deposit the medication in. So we measure a range of lengths – hence the need to add a prefix to denote whether we are describing a large or short length.

If we were trying to identify the size of a pressure-relieving mattress for a bed or the size of a dressing to cover a surgical wound, we would need to take two lengths into account, sometimes a longer length and shorter length (width), thus:

Length

Width

Dressings such as Melolin come in the following sizes: 5 cm × 5 cm, 10 cm × 10 cm and 10 cm × 20 cm. Sometimes we do not just want to know individual lengths (measurement of a to b), but we need to know the length *around* something, i.e. the perimeter or border (a to a).

Examples of measuring perimeter in health care include measuring girth (e.g. the waist), which is more accurately described as circumference. We also need to measure small circumferences,

Table 5.4 Summary of units of length

SI unit	Symbol	Value
kilometre	km	1,000 m
metre	m	1 m
centimetre	cm	$1/100$ m
millimetre	mm	$1/1,000$ m

such as the skull circumference of a neonate. The base unit of length is the metre.

Weight and mass

As mentioned above, often the measurements of height and weight are used together – for example, to establish that a new baby is developing normally or to establish a healthy weight for an adult.

Body mass index

Body mass index (BMI) is determined by comparing a patient's weight with their height. This allows us to identify whether a patient's health is at risk – if a patient is overweight or obese this will increase their risk of coronary heart disease. This measurement can be determined by dividing the weight (in kg) by the square of the person's height (in m^2). However, in practice most health care professionals use a chart. Figure 4.2 (in Chapter 4) is an example of this type of graph and is commonly used in health care.

Centile charts

The weight of a baby or young child can be plotted on a centile chart (sometimes called a percentile chart). This allows us to compare the baby's weight with other measurements in order to assess their growth and development. The other measurements considered are age, height (length) and head circumference. In other words, if we know a baby's weight and size (head circumference and length) at birth, using regular measurements we can establish whether the baby is growing at an appropriate rate.

These 'appropriate' physical milestones in a baby's development have been established using information collected about child development over a long period of time, so the centile chart uses an average weight for a baby of a certain size at a certain age for comparison purposes (these averages are the *centiles*).

Body surface area

Sometimes we take the measurement of weight on its own, for example on admission prior to elective (waiting list) surgery to establish a baseline for comparison after surgery, to calculate the dose of some medicines such as methotrexate (used commonly in rheumatoid arthritis), to promote healthy eating, or to establish the effectiveness of diuretic therapy in a patient with heart failure (discussed in more detail in Chapter 7).

More commonly, where the dose of a medicine needs to be carefully considered in relation to the individual patient's body size, for example in children, we use body surface area. This is usually achieved using a nomogram, a chart which has body surface area calculated based upon height and weight. According to Lapham and Agar (2003), this is based upon work undertaken by Du Bois and Du Bois in 1916, who carried out a series of measurements to establish the body surface area of a number of individuals. This means that in practice if we know the height and weight of a patient, we only have to consult the nomogram where all the calculations regarding body surface area are reproduced for us.

In health care, we tend to use the words 'mass' and 'weight' interchangeably, but there is a subtle difference in meaning between the two terms. Weight is dependent on the force of gravity pulling us down. So if the force of gravity alters, our weight will alter, even though our 'substance' has not changed. So the astronaut weighs less when he experiences the Moon's weaker gravitational pull and needs weighted boots to keep him on the surface of the Moon.

This 'substance' is referred to as *mass* and remains constant. So the more accurate way of referring to weight in clinical contexts is mass.

The gram is the unit for mass. Kilogram is the term used to describe a patient's weight – a larger amount – and milligram and microgram refer to the small amounts of 'substances', for example in medicines. Any medicine will contain the active ingredient, i.e. the drug. A medicine also contains other ingredients (excipients) which vary from manufacturer to manufacturer, for example flavourings and substances to speed up or slow down the absorption of the drug. All these excipients will be expressed in grams.

Another example of the use of grams in health care is in nutritional values. We may be worried about the amount of protein in the diet of a patient with chronic renal failure, and therefore the dietician may recommend a daily intake of no more than 0·6–0·8 grams per kilogram of the patient's body weight per day. It is important to note that this is an example and that patients' requirements would always be based upon an individual patient assessment (Whitney *et al.* 2001).

Amounts of substance

This measurement is concerned with laboratory tests such as those to determine substances contained or carried in the bloodstream, e.g. blood glucose in the patient with diabetes mellitus, or the constituents of fluids given intravenously, e.g. potassium.

The unit of substance is the mole. The mole refers to the mass (weight) of molecules or atoms that make up the formula of a compound such as glucose.

If a substance is dissolved or carried in a solution, we describe the amount present as the concentration. This is a derived unit, as it refers to the amount of the substance within an amount of fluid.

The normal range for a fasting blood glucose level is 3·5–5·5 mmol/litre; this means there are 3·5–5·5 mmol of glucose per litre of blood.

Patients returning from theatre who cannot tolerate oral fluids and diet may have their fluids and nutrients administered intravenously. A prescription you may be familiar with is that of sodium chloride 0·9%. We can interpret this as meaning there are 9 grams of sodium per litre.

Time

Some authors identify time as a unit used with SI units. While this in itself is not a vital piece of information, it does help to remind us that measurements of time are different from those we have used previously. For example, if you travel for 20 minutes on the first part of your journey, and after a break it takes 50 minutes to complete your journey, then the total journey time would be 70 minutes, which could also be expressed as 1 hour and 10 minutes. This reflects the fact that there are 60 minutes in an hour (if we were using the metric system we would expect there to be 100 minutes in an hour). An hour is made up of 60 minutes, and each minute is made up of 60 seconds. Therefore, there are 3,600 seconds (60 minutes × 60 seconds) in one hour. The unit of time is the second.

There are two ways of expressing time: the 12-hour clock and the 24-hour clock. When using the 12-hour clock we would use the terms a.m. and p.m. to denote what time of day we are referring to, e.g. 3 a.m. or 3 p.m. If we were using the 24-hour clock, we would refer to 03.00 hours and 15.00 hours. Most charts used within health care now reflect the 24-hour clock.

When using a 24-hour clock, 2.30 p.m. becomes 14.30 hours (i.e. we add 12 to 2.30). If we needed to translate the 24-hour clock when helping a patient to understand the time of their next appointment, 13.00 hours would become 1 p.m. (we subtract 12).

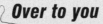
Over to you

Refresher – time

a. If an intravenous infusion of one litre sodium chloride commenced at 08.45 hours and finished at 13.50, how long has it taken to deliver the infusion?

State your answer in figures and words

b. Convert these times so that they refer to the 24-hour clock:

10.30 a.m.

10.30 p.m.

c. Convert these times from the 24-hour clock to a.m. or p.m.:

06.45

18.20

Derived units

In addition to the SI base units, there are *derived* units. These measurements are more complex and are made up of more than one base unit. For example, the unit of volume could be used to describe an amount of liquid in a glass that we need to record on a patient's fluid balance chart, the amount of blood being transfused from a bag, or the amount of a gas such as oxygen in a cylinder.

It is very difficult to capture this type of measurement, and in fact the unit of volume is *derived* from the units of length, breadth and height (see below).

Although there are many derived units, those used in health care are as shown in Table 5.5.

Volume

Volume is a measurement of capacity, e.g. the volume of milk in a bottle. The volume, or capacity, of a bottle refers to the amount it can hold. We cannot establish the amount of milk in the bottle solely

Table 5.5 Derived units

Quantity	SI unit	Symbol
Volume	litre	l
Energy	joule	J
Pressure	pascal	Pa
Temperature	kelvin	K

by measuring the height of the milk in the bottle, or the diameter of the bottle. The unit of volume is derived from the units of length, breadth and height, so we need to know all these measurements to find a volume.

The unit of volume is the litre. As with other units, we need to be able to describe small amounts, for example the amount of insulin contained in a cartridge for an insulin pen (3 ml), the amount of milk/formula in a baby's bottle (180 ml), or the amount of urine passed overnight into a leg bag (600 ml).

Medical gases such as oxygen and air are also measured in litres. A standard oxygen cylinder contains 1,360 litres of compressed gas (oxygen cylinders come in different sizes – this refers to a size F cylinder).

Temperature

The unit for temperature is the kelvin (K). However, in health care we use Celsius/centigrade as these measurements all record the same temperature interval (Bell 1993).

Recording a patient's temperature is often described as a *vital sign* or *clinical observation*. Normal body temperature is described as being approximately 37°C. The C refers to Celsius (also called centigrade); when recording temperature in a clinical area we usually refer to it as 'degrees centigrade'.

The 'normal' temperature range is from 36·2 °C to 37·7°C. The reason for identifying a range, as with other clinical observations, is that the normal body temperature fluctuates depending upon the time of day, and is usually higher in the evening. You could record the temperature of half a dozen patients in your care and find slight variations between them. Women trying to conceive take their temperature to identify when they are ovulating as temperature fluctuates over the course of a woman's menstrual cycle.

The range of temperature measurements identified above involve the use of a decimal point; decimals were discussed in Chapter 4.

We are able to maintain our body temperature within this 'normal' range despite fluctuations in, for example, the room temperature. However, sometimes, when the patient contracts an infection, or when the body is exposed to an extremely cold environment for a considerable length of time, for example, then our *thermoregulation mechanism* (Tortora and Grabowski 2003) may not be able to maintain the normal body temperature. Temperature in this context refers to the balance between the heat produced and acquired by the body (Marieb 2001). A patient might then become pyrexial (have a higher-than-normal body temperature) or hypothermic (have a low body temperature).

We may record skin temperature (using a clinical, electronic or disposable thermometer), temperature of the tympanic membrane (a tympanic thermometer uses infrared energy), or core temperature. Core temperature is the more accurate measurement and relates to 'the temperature of the organs within the cranial, thoracic and abdominal cavities' (Baillie 2005).

However, consider some other examples of temperature measurement that are important in clinical areas:

- The correct temperature to store medicines or blood products
- The temperature of the water in a bath for an older patient
- The need for a constant environmental temperature for premature babies.

Reflective activity

Can you think of any other examples of temperature measurement from your clinical area?

Energy

Probably the most useful and familiar example of energy measurement is in nutrition, when we use it to refer to how much food we need in order to be able to carry out our daily tasks/ recreation without either gaining or losing weight. A lot of us are familiar with this as calorie counting, comparing the calorific values of food based upon age, height and gender in order to avoid weight gain or to try to lose weight. Most diets also advocate taking exercise as this increases the amount of energy we use, so we use up our calories faster. The SI unit for energy is the joule *not* the calorie. As the joule (J) is a small unit, we usually use the kilojoule (kJ).

Pressure

Pressure (stress) is a derived unit. It can be expressed as 'the force per unit area' (James *et al.* 2002) and expressed thus:

$$\text{pressure} = \frac{\text{force}}{\text{area}}$$

The greater the area that a force is applied to, the smaller the pressure produced. For example, women wearing stiletto heels can damage floors such as laminates because all their force (or weight) is concentrated in a small area, whereas if someone wears trainers, the force is spread over a larger surface area and is therefore not as destructive.

Pressure as force over an area is demonstrated in the development of pressure ulcers. Whether the patient is sitting or lying, the tissues over bony prominences bear most of the weight. This leads to the development of pressure ulcers on the heels, sacrum and shoulders.

There are other examples of situations where pressure is important. If you think about using a hosepipe to water the garden you know that if the hose becomes blocked, the water will not be able to get through and the pressure in the hose will rise, sometimes with disastrous consequences.

Try to apply this to what you know about the sizes of wound drains, syringes, needles and the viscosity (thickness) of fluids travelling through these tubes. The thickness of the fluid and diameter of the tube will determine the amount of force to apply.

Nebulisers are another example of the application of pressure. Nebulisers are used for patients with respiratory problems. They provide a means of delivering a respiratory drug or medicine via a route that requires minimum effort from the patient. The nebuliser is a way of changing a liquid drug into droplet form that can then be inhaled by forcing it through a narrow opening under pressure. The pressure is usually provided by a pressurised gas such as air or oxygen, depending upon the patient's condition (James *et al.* 2002).

Pressure measurements in health care are recorded in different ways depending on what is being measured:

- Blood gases would be recorded using the pascal (Pa)
- Arterial blood pressure is recorded using mmHg.

Blood pressure

Blood pressure (BP) is one of the most important non-invasive observations that we record in practice. It is also carried out frequently, and decisions regarding a patient's treatment can be based upon one measurement or trends in BP measurement alone. It provides us with information about the health of the cardiovascular system, and is defined as 'the force or pressure which blood exerts on the walls of the blood vessels' (Baillie 2005). It is obtained from the volume of blood expelled from the heart with every beat/contraction (cardiac output), the volume of blood in the circulation (circulating blood volume) and the 'stretch' or elasticity of the walls of the blood vessels (peripheral resistance).

Two measurements are recorded:

- The systolic blood pressure, which is the force exerted when the ventricle contracts, and so is the maximum pressure of the blood against the artery wall
- The diastolic, which is said to reflect the pressure exerted on the arterial wall when the heart is at rest.

The two measurements are always considered together, and therefore constitute one measurement.

BP used to be measured with a mercury sphygmomanometer, which is no longer recommended due to concerns about the safety of mercury. However, because the method involved the health care professional studying a column of mercury to establish at what point on this column they could hear the systolic and diastolic pressures, it did help in visualising what was being recorded, i.e. a measurement of pressure. The use of a cuff, whether with a mercury sphygmomanometer or electronic monitoring device, can also help visualisation. The inflation of the cuff helps to remind us of the force being applied to the artery to temporarily stop the blood flow through it.

NB: The difference between the systolic and diastolic blood pressure is described as the *pulse pressure*, and like other observations this is important in clinical contexts as it indicates the health of the cardiovascular system.

Pulse

Recording a BP manually will involve palpating the patient's pulse. The patient's pulse rate is a good indicator of the health of the cardiovascular system. The pulse is a pressure wave of blood caused by the expansion and return (recoil) of the arteries as they accommodate blood pumped into the circulation by the heart beating (cardiac cycle). It is possible to determine some information about the heart beat/rate by measuring the pulse, for example at the wrist (radial pulse). We can also make judgements about the *quality* of the pulse, whether it is strong or weak. We count the pulse rate; this allows us to establish not only the rate but also the regularity of the heart. For example, sometimes the heart rate quickens and slows in relationship to the patient's rate of breathing, and this would be accepted as normal for that patient. However, when the patient has a fast heart rate as a consequence of disease or medications, the rate can often be irregular. When recording a pulse, it is important to record it for a whole minute. In practice, because of pressure on our time it is often tempting to record the pulse rate for quarter of a minute (15 seconds) and multiply by four. If we do this and the heart rate is irregular, it will only reflect the heart rate for 15 instead of 60 seconds, and an incorrect measurement could result. Also, if the heart rate is irregular, the weaker beats may not be felt at the wrist because of its distance from the heart, so the better pulse to record is the *apical* pulse, i.e. a stethoscope is placed on the chest and positioned over the apex of the heart to record the heart rate. If a patient's heart rate is altered, there is usually a comparative alteration in their blood pressure, i.e. if a patient is bleeding heavily after an accident, their blood pressure will drop because of the decreasing blood volume due to the blood loss, while their heart rate will increase as the heart beats faster to maintain the circulation.

So clinical measurements such as blood pressure, pulse rate and temperature are often considered together.

Over to you

Identify three clinical situations where the overall picture of observations is considered.

You might have identified shock, monitoring reactions to blood transfusions and neurological observations.

To sum up, the physical quantities we measure frequently in health care are:

- Length
- Mass
- Amounts of substance
- Volume
- Temperature
- Energy
- Pressure.

However, these measurements are meaningless unless we understand why we are measuring them, and the impact they have on patient care.

Conclusions

This chapter has introduced you to the SI units in health care together with some clinical examples of the relevance of these to patient care. We have offered some examples of how to calculate using SI units and identified situations where these units are considered together, for example, to determine the health status of patients.

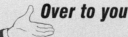

Over to you

Refresher – SI units

A patient is to receive an injection of cimetidine 120 mg by the intramuscular route. Ampoules on hand contain 200 mg/2 ml

a. To what do the terms mg and ml refer?

b. Calculate the dose required

A patient is prescribed 0·06 grams of codeine phosphate. Tablets on the ward contain 30 mg

a. How many milligrams are there in a gram?

b. Which unit of measurement has the gram as its SI unit?

c. Convert the 0·06 grams into mg

d. Calculate the dose required

A boy is to receive an intravenous infusion of 400 ml glucose over eight hours. The barrel emits 60 drops per ml

a. To what does the abbreviation ml refer?

b. Calculate the correct drip rate in drops per minute

A child is prescribed Erythromycin. He is to receive 50 mg per kg of body weight per day, which is to be split into four doses. The child weighs 12 kg

a. To what does the abbreviation kg refer?

b. Work out the daily dose for this child

c. Work out the individual dose for this child

A child is prescribed Digoxin elixir 0·08 mg. The stock solution contains 0·05 mg per ml

a. How many micrograms are contained in a milligram?

b. Convert the 0·08 mg and the 0·05 mg to micrograms

c. Which unit of measurement has the millilitre as its SI unit?

d. Work out an individual dose of Digoxin for this child

A patient is prescribed 150 micrograms of levothyroxine. On hand are 0·05 mg tablets

a. To what does the abbreviation mg refer?

b. Work out the dose to be given

A patient is to receive an intravenous infusion of 1 litre of sodium chloride 0.98% over eight hours

a. How many millilitres in a litre?

b. Calculate the drip rate required in drops per minute (the drop factor is 20)

A patient is prescribed 9 mg of morphine intramuscularly. The ampoule contains 15 mg in 1 ml

a. Work out the correct dose

Phenobarbitone 60 mg has been ordered. Stock ampoules contain 200 mg/ml.

a. What volume should be given?

> ## RRRRRRapid recap
>
> Check your progress so far by working through each of the following points
> 1. What do SI units denote?
> 2. What is meant by the term 'derived' unit?
> 3. Why have SI units been adopted?
> 4. Give three prefixes which would be used to denote a small unit
>
> If you have difficulty with more than one of the questions, read through the section again to refresh your understanding before moving on.

References

Baillie, L. (ed.) (2005) *Developing Nursing Skills*. Hodder Arnold, London.

Bell, R.J. (ed.) (1993) *The International System of Units*, 6th edn. National Physical Library, HMSO, London.

Coben, D. and Atere-Roberts, E. (2005) *Calculations for Nursing and Healthcare*, 2nd edn. Palgrave Macmillan, Hampshire.

Gregory, S. (2002) Writing a prescription. *Practice Nurse*, **25**(4), 24–26.

Hutton, B.M. (2003) Calculations for new prescribers. *Nursing Standard*, **17**(25), 47–53.

James, J., Baker, C. and Swain, H. (2002) *Principles of Science for Nurses*. Blackwell Science Ltd, Oxford.

Kapborg, I.D. (1994) An Evaluation of Swedish nurse students' calculation ability in relation to their earlier educational background. *Nurse Education today*, **15**, 69–74.

Lapham, R. and Agar, H. (2003) *Drug Calculations for Nurses. A Step-by-Step Approach*, 2nd edn. Arnold, Great Britain.

Less cholesterol, www.lesscholesterol.co.uk.

Marieb, E. (2001) *Human Anatomy and Physiology*, 5th edn. Benjamin Cummings, San Francisco.

NHS Estates (2003) *Infection Control in the Built Environment: Design and Planning*, 2nd edn. Department of Health, London.

Tortora, G.J. and Grabowski, S.R. (2003) *Principles of Anatomy and Physiology*, 10th edn. Wiley, New York.

Whitney, E.N., Cataldo, C.B., Debruyne, L.K. and Rolfes, S.R. (2001) *Nutrition for Health and Health Care*, 2nd edn. Wadsworth.

Wikipedia, www.en.wikipedia.org.

Woodrow, P. (1998) Numeracy skills. *Nursing Standard*, **12**(30), 48–53.

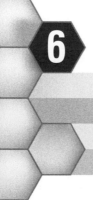

6 Applying theory to practice: explaining and unpacking our approach to nursing numeracy

Learning outcomes

By the end of this chapter you should be able to:

- Identify strategies to help you manage number problems successfully

- Describe our approach to nursing numeracy

- Start to apply this approach to number problems within care settings

- Identify some examples of numeracy in nursing

This chapter pulls together issues identified within previous chapters, such as maths anxiety, difficulty in identifying where we use numbers in nursing, and strategies for 'managing' numbers. We revisit them in order to introduce you to our approach to identifying, and strategies for working with, numbers within nursing contexts. Chapters 7 to 10 develop these strategies and apply them to specific and individual patient case studies. We want to take you on a journey, starting from perceived problems or concerns about your numeracy performance, and take you from this concern to solutions. Figure 6.1 clarifies this, but each aspect is explained in more detail below.

Numeracy difficulties

There are many reasons for numeracy difficulties. Some of these reasons are explored in Chapter 2 to help you to identify the cause of your difficulties so that you can address it and become competent and confident in your number skills.

It seems that nursing is considered a feminine profession (Davies 1998) and this has had advantages and disadvantages. Nursing is not perceived to require scientific knowledge and, as a result, nurses are pictured as having little or no use for numbers in their daily work nor having the requirement of number skills. The one exception is where nurses use number skills in their daily work to calculate doses of medicines. However, many nurses are not involved in administering medicines on a daily basis but are still involved with daily calculations. If we are confronted with unexpected calculations in busy clinical areas, it can be difficult to consider the numeracy problem and identify strategies to solve the problem.

Numeracy difficulties together with the complex nature of care

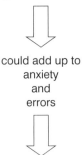

could add up to
anxiety
and
errors

We want to change this to positive outcomes/solutions

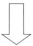

We have therefore developed a series of steps

1. Identify where the numbers and therefore numeracy appears in nursing care
2. Consider how we 'think' about number
3. Build upon existing skills and use the work of mathematical experts
4. Use tools/strategies effectively.

Those we identify and use in the following chapters are:
- **Skills checklist**
- **Theory and practice**
- **Top tips**

Figure 6.1 *Our approach to nursing numeracy*

The complex nature of care

Contemporary nursing is both complex and dynamic. Changing technologies, higher patient expectations and government drivers frequently seem to be influencing developments (DOH 2002; NHS Plan 2000). This means that qualified nurses are expected to take on even more skills, such as diagnosis, managing patient caseloads and running clinics. Patients who are more dependent are nursed in increasingly technological environments. Treatments are becoming more complex; patients are prescribed multiple medicines in order to combat multipathology. The genome project has opened up the possibility of more genetic therapies. Added to this, our patients are becoming active partners in their care, better informed and requiring information from health care workers to enable them to make informed decisions.

Numeracy anxiety

Past experience may have made us very negative about our numeracy skills. Chapter 2 explored the complex reasons that underpin this. Whatever the reasons for our perceived weaknesses, it appears that we may be guilty of persuading ourselves that we cannot do sums, as confidence has a direct bearing on our competence.

Errors

Despite increasing knowledge and developing nurses' roles, the rate of medicine errors is increasing. There are many reasons for this, such as busy clinical environments, but Trim (2004) suggests that nurses have difficulties with the mathematical, conceptual and measurement elements of the calculation.

Positive outcomes/solutions

Identifying where the numeracy in nursing is

Traditional approaches to teaching calculation skills seem to be successful only in the short term. There are several potential explanations for this: numeracy generates anxiety and clinical areas are busy and demanding. Also, most texts focus on the teaching of calculation related to medicines and intravenous infusion. However, with the development of specialist nursing roles, nurses need to be competent in number skills within a range of contexts, for example, staffing levels, patient education, interpreting evidence and carrying out risk assessment, and these seem to apply to a range of care environments. In order to help you visualise where numeracy occurs in nursing, we have identified the elements that seem to be common to all nursing roles: care management, resource management and risk management. Although the elements that have been identified within each of these component parts for the purpose of this book are focused on nursing, this model can be used to represent any area of practice. Set out below are individual examples of numeracy within each of these categories and we will go on to explore and develop these within the four patient care studies in Chapters 7 to 10. These ideas are also presented as a diagram (see Figure 6.2).

Consider how we think about number

We enter nursing programmes with a wealth of life experience which means that we have also learnt how to carry out calculations.

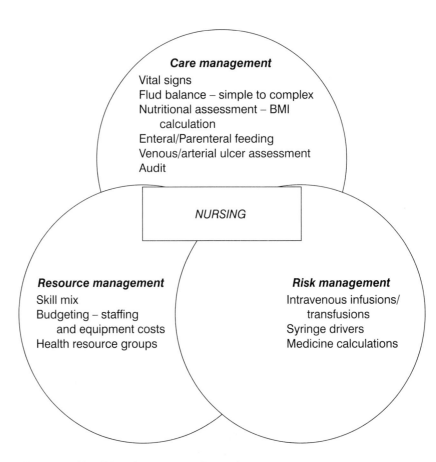

Figure 6.2 *Identifying the numeracy in nursing*

Some of us are good at mental arithmetic but often cannot explain how we achieved the answer. Others like to approach problems in a linear way, using a series of steps and working through the problem logically (Chinn 1998). The fact that we achieve answers in different ways is unimportant, but sometimes we may feel that other ways work better. Chapter 4 introduced you to some strategies for undertaking calculation, but these are not the only ways to tackle number problems.

There have been changes to mathematics teaching in schools as mathematical experts try to solve the conundrum of the most effective way of enabling students to learn. BODMAS is a good example of this. This concept was discussed in Chapter 4 as an approach to tackling the elements of a number problem in the correct sequence. *BBC KS3 Bitesize Revision* (Kearsley Bullen 2003) identifies BODMAS as referring to Brackets, pOwers/roots, Division, Multiplication, Addition and Subtraction. Some of us were taught in school that this referred to Brackets *Of*, Division, Multiplication, Addition and Subtraction. Other authors refer to BEDMAS: Brackets, Exponentiation (another way of referring to powers), Division, Multiplication, Addition and Subtraction (Lapham and Agar 2003). These differences in themselves are not important, but they do need to be recommended by a credible source and they need to be successful. What is important is that you understand how you achieved your answer and can verify it in some way. Also, you need to recognise which methods work for you because they suit your thinking/learning style. The strategies outlined below are intended to help you get there.

Build upon existing skills and use the work of mathematical experts

Some authors (Ollerton 2003) suggest that solving mathematical problems is about applying a set of rules or strategies, usually a combination of strategies. However, Pólya (1990) felt that this would not promote the transferability of skills and therefore adopted a problem-solving approach to enable his students to use and build on previous experience. We have modified this approach to show other elements such as reflection and your professional development. The 'tool' that we use to put the number skills into the context of nursing work in the following pages is called the Skills checklist. You will see this and other strategies appear throughout the chapters containing the patient case studies to demonstrate how they can be used.

Identifying and using the tools

The Skills checklist looks like this.

Skills checklist

The number skills required in this calculation are . . .
If you have been unable to do this or if you have had difficulty in doing this, ask yourself:

- Did I understand what I was being asked to do?
- Were there any number principles/formulae I could have used?

Perform the calculation and ask yourself:

- Is it correct?
- How did I feel about the process?
- What do I need to do now?

Key points **Top tips**

Within the Top tips boxes are reminders of the key points or 'tricks' to help you solve a specific numeracy problem.

Theory to practice

We have already identified that being asked to calculate in relation to a situation you have not had previous experience of is very difficult. This is because you have no reliable checking method within your experience to guide either the process or the answer. There is a strong argument in the preceding chapters for the learning to be contextualised; you might be getting the answers wrong because you do not understand the clinical condition, medications etc. Within these theory to practice boxes we identify some clinical information and refer you to useful sources of information.

How to use the following chapters

In order to help you to recognise where numeracy skills are in nursing and to develop your numeracy skills, the remaining chapters of this book explore some patient scenarios/case studies. We have chosen to include four particular patient case studies as they represent some very commonly occurring situations that many nurses will be familiar with. These case studies will enable you to take part in a variety of activities that will help you to identify where your strengths lie, and if you have any areas of weakness, where these areas are.

RRRRRRapid recap

Check your progress so far by working through each of the following points

1. Name the three elements of care inherent in the approach to nursing numeracy used here
2. Identify the strategies used in the approach in this book
3. Explain why the approach in this book fosters transferability of learning
4. Discuss the benefits of this approach for your professional development.

If you have difficulty with more than one of the questions, read through the section again to refresh your understanding before moving on.

References

BBC GCSE Bitesize Revision, www.bbc.co.uk/schools/gcsebitesize.

Chinn, S. (1998) *Sum Hope. Breaking the Numbers Barrier*. Souvenir Press, London.

Davies, C. (1998) *Gender and the Professional Predicament in Nursing*. Open University Press, Buckingham.

Department of Health (2000) *The NHS Plan*. Department of Health, London.

Department of Health (2002) *Developing Key Roles For Nurses And Midwives: A Guide For Managers*. Department of Health, London.

Kearsley Bullen, R. (2003) *BBC KS3 Bitesize Revision*. BBC worldwide, England. See also www.bbc.co.uk/bitesize.

Lapham, R. and Agar, H. (2003) *Drug Calculations for Nurses. A Step-by-Step Approach*, 2nd edn. Arnold.

Ollerton, M. (2003) *Getting the Buggers to Add Up*. Continuum, London.

Pólya, G. (1990) *How to Solve It: A New Aspect of Mathematical Method*, 2nd edn. Penguin, London.

Trim, J. (2004) Clinical skills: a practical guide to working out drug calculations. *British Journal of Nursing*, **13**(10), 602–607.

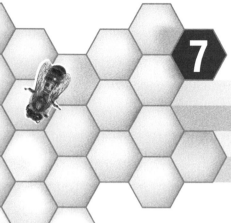

7 Exploring the nursing numeracy skills embedded in caring for a patient in the community:

Mr Aurek Dabrowski

Learning outcomes

By the end of this chapter you should be able to:

- Recognise where numbers are in the nursing care of patients such as Aurek Dabrowski
- Calculate in a variety of nursing-related contexts
- Use numeracy skills to explore the nursing care of Mr Dabrowski

Introduction

In order to explore some of the numeracy skills embedded in caring for patients in a critical care setting, this chapter introduces you to Mr Aurek Dabrowski.

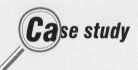

Case study

Aurek Dabrowski

Aurek Dabrowski is a 73-year-old ex-publican. Nearly three years ago he visited his GP complaining of short periods of rapid heartbeats and feeling dizzy. He is widowed and lives with his partner of eight months, Emily, in a two-bedroom flat on the second floor of a building near the town centre. He has a son who lives in Australia. He and Emily both try to follow the advice they were given about eating healthily. However, while he did stop smoking for about two years, Aurek began again about six months ago, but says 'he only smokes when he is out having a drink or two'. He acknowledges calling in for a drink or two every day. During this visit to the surgery the GP noted that Aurek's BP was 150/80mmHg, pulse rate 88bpm regular rhythm, height 1·82 metres and weight 82 kg. His ECG revealed sinus rhythm.

Normal ECG tracing paper runs through most ECG machines at a set rate and is marked in large and small squares so that the time between each part of the cardiac cycle can be measured. Each large square represents 0·2 seconds, while each small square represents

0·04 seconds. As a result, there are 300 large squares per minute. There are 60 seconds in a minute, so you will have to divide 60 by 0·2:

$$\frac{60}{0.2} = 300$$

to confirm this.

So, *as long as the patient's heart rate is regular*, you can count the number of large squares between each QRS complex and divide that number into 300 to give the approximate heart rate – e.g. if there are six large squares between each QRS complex the approximate heart rate would be:

$$\frac{300}{6} = 50 \text{ beats per minute}$$

As long as the heart rate on the ECG tracing is regular, you can make an approximate calculation of heart rate by counting the large squares between each QRS complex.

Over to you

Care management

Below is part of the ECG trace taken at Aurek's last visit to the practice nurse. From the ECG tracing below, estimate Aurek's approximate heart rate.

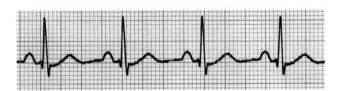

Figure 7.1 *Aurek's ECG trace*

There are approximately four large squares between each of the QRS complexes (a part of the waveform representation of the electrical activity of the heart on an ECG) in the above ECG tracing, so your answer will be 75. If you have not got this answer, check your calculations again. If you are using a calculator, check your data entry carefully to make sure you have keyed in the correct numbers. Most incorrect answers when using a calculator are caused by operator error. If you have keyed in the correct numbers and your calculations are still not giving you the right answer, are you sure that you have divided 300 by 4? Your calculation should look like this:

$$\frac{300}{4} = 75$$

Key points **Top tips**

When using calculators in clinical areas, get into the habit of checking carefully each set of numbers that you key in. Remember the old adage 'Rubbish in, rubbish out'.

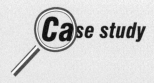
Case study

Case study continued

About two months ago, Aurek noticed that he seemed to be rather breathless when he was walking, particularly up steps, slopes and inclines. Thinking this meant that he needed to become a bit fitter, he set himself a goal to walk 10,000 steps a day and even bought himself a pedometer. However, he found it very difficult to achieve his goal and as he was mostly only managing around 3,000 steps a day, he stopped using the pedometer. For the last two or three weeks he has also tried to cut down his food intake as he noticed that his trousers were getting tighter around the waist. Although he was not conscious of it, Emily noticed that Aurek was wearing trainers most of the time rather than the shoes he really preferred. Emily thought this was because his feet were swollen and his trainers were more comfortable as he could adjust the laces. On Saturday, while shopping, Emily noticed that Aurek was breathless by the time they stopped for coffee. Aurek also had a dull ache in his chest which happened from time to time, but he thought it could not be serious as it always went away when he stopped moving around. He had not mentioned it to Emily as he did not want her to worry. She suggested that he should get himself checked out if only for her sake. On Monday, at Aurek's request, Emily rang the surgery and made an appointment for him to have a check-up. During the appointment with the practice nurse, Aurek's assessment included BP, pulse, CLASP (Cardiovascular Limitations And Symptoms Profile) score, ECG (electrocardiogram) and BMI (Body Mass Index) score. Aurek's BP was 150/85mmHg, pulse rate 122bpm irregular rhythm, height 1·82 metres and weight 91·5 kg. His ECG revealed atrial fibrillation. Aurek completed the following chart so that the practice nurse could calculate his CLASP score.

Cardiovascular Limitations and Symptoms Profile (CLASP score)

Angina

A1   On average, how often have you had angina in the last 2 weeks?
Once or twice a week, but not every day	1
2 to 3 times a week, but not every day	②
Once a day	3
2–3 times a day	4
4 or more times a day	5

A2   On average, over the last 2 weeks, how intense have your episodes of angina been?
Mostly mild	1
Mostly moderate	②
Mostly severe	3

A3   Has angina woken you up at night in the last 2 weeks?
Not at all	1
Occasionally	②
Often	3
Very often	4

A4   With respect to your angina, in the last 2 weeks have you had:
Mostly good days?	1
Good and bad days?	②
Only bad days?	3

A5   Overall, how bad has your angina been over the last 2 years?
Mild	1
Moderate	②
Severe	3

Shortness of breath

B1   On average, how often have you been short of breath in the last 2 weeks?
Once or twice in the last fortnight	1
2 to 3 times a week, but not every day	1
Once a day	2
2–3 times a day	3
4 or more times a day	③

B2   Have you found it difficult to lie flat without becoming short of breath?
Not at all	1
A little	2
A moderate amount	3
A great deal	③

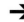

Figure 7.2 *Mr Dabrowski's completed CLASP score (2006, reproduced under licence)*
Source: National Service Framework for Coronary Heart Disease *(Department of Health 2000) Chapter 6, Heart Failure. Department of Health. Crown copyright material is reproduced with the permission of the Controller of HMSO and the Queen's Printer for Scotland*

B3 With respect to your shortness of breath in the last 2 weeks, have you had:

Mostly good days?	1
Good and bad days?	②
Only bad days?	2

B4 Overall, how bad has your shortness of breath been over the last 2 weeks?

Mild	1
Moderate	②
Severe	3

B5 How much has your shortness of breath interfered with your life over the last 2 weeks?

Not at all	1
A little	1
A moderate amount	②
A great deal	3

Ankle swelling

C1 How swollen have your ankles been in the last 2 weeks?

Slightly swollen	1
Moderately swollen	2
Very swollen	③

C2 Overall, how bad has your ankle swelling been over the last 2 weeks?

Mild	1
Moderate	②
Severe	3

C3 How much has your ankle swelling interfered with your life over the last 2 weeks?

Not at all	1
A little	2
A moderate amount	③
A great deal	4

Cardiovascular Limitations and Symptoms Profile (CLASP) score

Interpretation

Individual questions are scored and summed to give totals for each dimension of the questionnaire: angina, shortness of breath and ankle swelling.

Within each of these totals, threshold scores are provided to classify clients as mild, moderate or severe, depending on the level of impairment or level of functioning.

Figure 7.2 *continued*

Angina	Questions A1–A5
Total	5–17
Mild	5–8
Moderate	9–12
Severe	13–17

Consider referral if your symptoms are new or deteriorating, or if your score is 10 or more.

Shortness of breath	Questions B1–B5
Total	5–14
Mild	5–7
Moderate	8–10
Severe	11–14

Consider referral if your symptoms are new or deteriorating, or if your score is 9 or more.

Ankle swelling	Questions C1–C3
Total	3–10
Mild	3–4
Moderate	5–7
Severe	8–10

Consider referral if your symptoms are new or deteriorating, or if your score is 8 or more.

Figure 7.2 *continued*

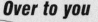

Over to you

Care management

From Aurek's completed CLASP chart above, identify his CLASP score.

Aurek's CLASP score is angina: 5 (mild); shortness of breath: 12 (severe); ankle swelling: 8 (severe). The *National Service Framework for Coronary Heart Disease* (Department of Health 2000, Chapter 6) suggests that with a CLASP score like this, Aurek should be referred to specialist services rather than being managed in the community.

Theory to practice

Working in situations such as this you need to be able to both collate and interpret numerical data.
● The CLASP data attempts to quantify how someone's symptoms are affecting their life
● The greater the score, the more the effects are felt by the patient and the more urgency there is to begin treatment.

Skills checklist

The number skill required in this calculation is addition. If you have been unable to do this calculation or you have had difficulty with it, ask yourself:

● Did I understand what I was being asked to do?

● Did I have the number skills to carry out this calculation?

● If you are having difficulty understanding the problem, is it because you have literacy problems such as dyslexia? There is a link between literacy problems and numeracy difficulties. There is also a much less common condition similar to dyslexia but it is difficulty with numbers rather than words. This condition is known as dyscalculia. If you know that you have dyslexia there is a useful book, Anne Henderson's (1998) *Maths for the Dyslexic*. If you suspect that you may have dyslexia, there are a number of places that you can get advice and assistance including the following resources:

learndirect have a website that explores dyslexia and numeracy: www.ufi.com/dyslexia/numeracy/implications.html.
The British Dyslexia Association web pages all about dyslexia may be useful: www.bdadyslexia.org.uk. They also have some helpful advice about dyscalculia as well as dyslexia and maths. This is available at www.bdadyslexia.org.uk/dyscalculia.html.
You may also find that the BBC Skillswise website has a helpful section about dyscalculia: www.bbc.co.uk/skillswise/tutors/expertcolumn/dyscalculia/index.shtml.

● Were there any number principles/formulae I could have used?

Perform the calculation and ask yourself:

● Is it correct?

● How did I feel about the process?

● What do I need to do now?

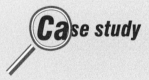

Case study continued

As the practice nurse is concerned about Aurek's condition, she refers him to his GP for an urgent appointment. During this consultation Aurek is diagnosed with heart failure and is prescribed furosemide (frusemide) 40 mg daily and Digoxin 125 mcg. In order to establish the effectiveness of the newly prescribed medication, the GP asks the practice nurse to weigh Aurek weekly.

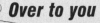

Over to you

Care management

Aurek's weight when he began his medication was 91·5 kg. Over the past four weeks his weight chart looks like this:

7/4/06   89·4 kg
14/4/06   88 kg
21/4/06   87·7 kg
28/4/06   86·5 kg

Calculate how much weight Aurek has lost. If one litre of water weighs one kg, how much fluid does this represent?

Subtracting Aurek 's final weight (86·5 kg) from his original weight before taking frusemide (91·5 kg) means that Aurek has lost 5 kg. Your written calculation would look like this: 91·5 – 86·5 = 5. As 1 litre of water weighs approximately 1 kg, this represents a fluid loss of 5 litres.

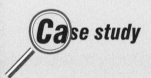

Case study

Case study continued

Aurek tells you that he feels much better and is keen to know how much weight he has lost in total, but he also wants to know this in imperial measurements.

Reflective activity

Think about how comfortable you feel explaining to patients and/or their carers how to calculate. If you feel uncomfortable about it, think about the strategies you can use to change how you feel. Could you use this learning opportunity in your Professional Portfolio?

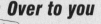

Over to you

Care management

Convert Aurek's weight loss (5 kg) to stones and pounds so that you can tell him how much weight he has lost.

If you have remembered that there are approximately 2·2 lb in a kg, your calculation will look like this: $(5 \times 2.2) = 11$. The answer has to be given in pounds – Aurek has lost 11 lb.

Theory to practice

Working in situations such as this, you need to understand what heart failure is and the impact it can have on both the patient and their family. Understanding what the treatment and management is trying to achieve will enable you to set the numeracy in context.

Heart failure is defined in the *National Service Framework* (NSF) *for Coronary Heart Disease* (Department of Health 2000) as 'a clinical syndrome caused by the heart's inability to pump blood around the body'. It goes on to say that 'most cases of heart failure are due to coronary heart disease and about a third result from hypertensive heart disease' (Chapter 6, p. 2).

Body mass index (BMI) assesses the relationship between two measurements: weight and height. Using this relationship, it is possible to establish at what point the person is on a scale. The scale identifies a range of suitable and unsuitable height to weight ratios in an attempt to highlight a healthy weight range or a range that may put someone at greater risk of weight-related disorders, e.g. type 2 diabetes.

◯━ *Keywords*
....

Formula

This is mathematical shorthand, rather like a recipe for calculating something. Following the instructions will ensure that you can carry out the calculation. However, be careful that when you do the calculation you do it in the correct order. Remember BODMAS if you are not sure what this is (see Chapter 4, p. 52)

Over to you

Care management

Which two measurements do you need to use to determine someone's body mass index?

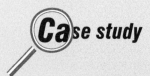
Case study

Case study continued

The practice nurse prefers to calculate BMI rather than rely on having a pre-printed scale to hand. She has found that people borrow the charts and never return them. When the practice nurse calculates Aurek's BMI, she uses the recognised **formula**, which is:

Weight (kg) ÷ Height (m²) = BMI

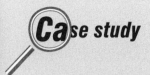

Case study

So, in order to use the above formula to calculate Aurek's BMI, you need to follow these three steps:

1. Find the height of the patient in metres and their weight in kg.
2. Multiply the figure for the height (in metres) by itself (this will give you the height squared): 1.82×1.82 m $= 3.31$ m^2.
3. Divide the weight (in kg) by the height squared (the answer you had in step two): 86.5 kg $\div 3.31$ m$^2 = 26.13$ kg/m^2.

(NB: If you do not have the patient's height and weight in metric measurements you may have the imperial measurements. These will need to be converted to metric measurements before you proceed to calculate the BMI. If you have to convert from imperial weight to metric, many people use 1 kg as being equivalent to 2.2 lb.)

Over to you

Care management

The ranges for BMI are as follows:
Men: 20.5–25.0
Women: 19–24
Overweight: 25–30
Obese: over 30
Underweight: less than 19

Tick which of the categories below that indicate that Aurek's BMI score of 26.13 suggests he is:

- Extremely obese
- Underweight
- Ideal weight
- Morbidly obese
- Obese
- Overweight.

A BMI score of 26.13 would suggest that Aurek is overweight. The Department of Health recommends that for people with a BMI of over 25, losing 5–10% of body weight will give considerable health benefits (www.dh.gov.uk).

Theory to practice

Working in situations such as this you need to understand:

- The advantages and disadvantages of using BMI
- The purpose of using an assessment of health risk based on body weight

The use of waist measurement is now also being advocated because of an increasing understanding of metabolic syndrome and its link to the risk of developing heart disease, hypertension and type 2 diabetes (Nigam *et al.* 2005). In an effort to include this current thinking it is now recommended by the Department of Health that you consider body shape and waist measurement in addition to weight and BMI when assessing patients (www.food.gov.uk). You might also find this a useful website to refer patients to. They may find the body shape information useful and also the general information about healthy eating.

Key points **Top tips**

- It is important for your personal and professional development that you use the Skills checklists. If you are having difficulty with any of the calculations they will help you to recognise and nurture the skills that you need. If you do not use this kind of structured approach to your learning, it may be difficult for you to identify which skills you should work on. For most people, time is a very precious commodity and using this sort of approach to learning uses time much more efficiently as it focuses on developing the skills needed, not on developing skills that you already have. The Skills checklist will help you to develop the numeracy skills that you need for practice. Once you have identified where you are having problems with numbers, you can then move forward and acquire the necessary skills.

- If you find that you need more help to develop any of your numeracy skills, you may like to identify this and your action plan in your Professional Portfolio and use one or more of the following resources to gain the skill that you need. This could then be recorded as professional development in your portfolio. While the following resources are not set in a nursing context they are useful distance learning resources that can help you learn the basic skills of addition, multiplication, division, fractions and decimals that once learnt can be transferred to nursing. Once you have these skills you should return to this book and complete the activities that you were having difficulty with. This will assure you that you can transfer the number skills you have learnt and it will also enable you to confirm your professional development in your portfolio. The two resources that you may find helpful are www.bbc.co.uk/schools/gcsebitesize and www.learndirect.org.uk.

The *National Service Framework for Coronary Heart Disease* (Department of Health 2000) states that 'the incidence of heart failure is about one new case per 1,000 population per year and is rising at about 10% per year' (Chapter 6, p. 2). This increasing incidence of heart failure will impact on the services provided. It is therefore important that consideration is given to this potential increase in service users and appropriate plans are made to provide services that will be able to meet any increased demand.

Over to you

Resource management

If you work in a city with a population of approximately 350,000, and given the statistics specified by the NSF above, how many new cases of heart failure will be seen in the next year?

Well done if you said that the answer is 350.

You may have been able to see straightaway in your head that the answer is 350.

Reflective activity

If you could not see that the answer is 350, think about what you were asked to do. Can you see what the problem is?

The question asks you to identify how much larger the city's population is than the 'per 1,000 population' cited by the NSF. The population is 350 times larger. Therefore, to work out the answer you have to divide the city population total by one new case per thousand (1,000). Mathematically, the calculation would look like this:

$$\frac{350,000}{1,000}$$

As with all calculations that involve units of tens, hundreds and thousands, you can cross out the noughts evenly on each of the figures. This would mean cancelling out the three noughts in the figure 1,000 and three of the noughts in the figure 350,000. This leaves 350 as the answer.

Skills checklist

The number skill asked for in this calculation is division. If you were unable to do this calculation or if you had difficulty doing the calculation ask yourself:

● Did I understand what I was being asked to do?
● Did I have the number skills to carry out this calculation?
● Were there any number principles/formulae I could have used?

Perform the calculation. Ask yourself:

● Is it correct?
● How did I feel about the process?
● What do I need to do now?

Key points | Top tips

Mathematics is about balance, therefore:

● Always make units of measurement the same on each side of the equation
● Equal numbers of noughts can be cancelled out at each side as well as at the top and bottom of each equation
● Everything that you do to the top part of a equation must be done to the bottom part of the equation.

Over to you

Resource management

As most of the people predicted to develop heart failure in the locality will be admitted to the Emergency Care Unit at some point over the next year, what concerns would this potential increase in patients stimulate in the senior staff?

The senior staff will be considering how they will meet this increased demand by exploring whether they have extra resources in:

● Bed occupancy rates
● Equipment and medicine budgets
● Staffing budget.

Or it may be that **re-engineering** the provision of services to people both in heart failure and those at risk of developing heart failure would provide a more patient focused, efficient and cost-effective service.

Keywords

Re-engineering
Used by large organisations such as the NHS to mean rearranging or reorganising service delivery

After cancelling out the noughts in the equation above, you are left with 350. This means that GP surgeries and a hospital in a town such as this should expect to have at least 350 new cases of heart failure in the next year.

The NSF goes on to state that the male to female **ratio** of patients developing heart failure is two to one. This is often written as 2:1. This means that for every female developing heart failure, there will be two men who acquire it.

> ## Over to you
>
> **Resource management**
>
> Given that the male to female ratio is 2:1, how many of the 350 predicted new cases of heart failure will be male and how many will be female?

Congratulations if you said that 233 new cases will be male and 117 new cases will be female. You were being asked to divide by three and then to multiply by two. The calculation would look like this:

$$\frac{350}{3} = 116\cdot66\ldots, \text{ or rounded up} = 117$$

So 117 will be the number of new female cases.

As the ratio of male to female is 2:1, you then have to multiply 116·66. . . by 2 (116·66 . . . × 2) to give the new male cases = 233·33 . . ., which rounds down to 233. To check that the sum of the two results is 350 the two answers should be added together: 117 + 233 = 350.

> ### Skills checklist
>
> The number skills required in this calculation are division and multiplication, as well as rounding up and down. If you have been unable to do this calculation or if you have had difficulty doing it, ask yourself:
>
> ●   Did I understand what I was being asked to do?
>
> ●   Did I have the number skills to carry out this calculation?
>
> ●   Were there any number principles/formulae I could have used?
>
> Perform the calculation. Ask yourself:
>
> ●   Is it correct?
>
> ●   How did I feel about the process?
>
> ●   What do I need to do now?

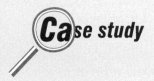

Case study continued

At Aurek's next review with the practice nurse, Aurek is complaining of frequent bouts of nausea, some anorexia and slightly blurred vision. His repeat ECG and vital signs show a bradycardia. As part of his clinical management plan she reduces his prescription for Digoxin from 125 micrograms to 62·5 micrograms. How will she explain this to Aurek?

The practice nurse will have to explain to Aurek that he is probably having too large a dose of Digoxin and that he would feel much better if he took a reduced dose. She will help him to understand that the dose that he should take from now is 62·5 micrograms – that is half the dose that he has been taking. The nurse will reassure him that if he does this, his symptoms should gradually stop. He will be advised to return to the surgery if they do not.

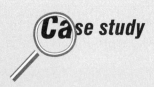

Case study continued

During his next visit to see the practice nurse, Aurek is asked about his understanding of the dietary advice that has been given to him in the past. As the Department of Health now recommends that an adult should eat no more than 6 grams of salt a day (www.salt.gov.uk), the practice nurse is particularly keen that Aurek understands about the salt content of food.

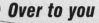

> ## Over to you
>
> **Care management**
> In order to check Aurek's understanding of how to calculate sodium content, the practice nurse shows him a label from a tin of low-salt, low-sugar baked beans and asks him to calculate how much salt there is in each portion of baked beans. The label reads 0·2 g sodium per 100 g. The tin size is 420 g and there are two portions in the tin (NB: salt content equals sodium content × 2·5). What should Aurek's answer be?

Aurek's answer should be 1·05 g of salt per portion. To calculate the correct answer, first you need to find out how many grams there are in a single portion of beans. Therefore, divide the tin size by 2, as there are two portions in the tin. This would give you 210 g (420 g ÷ 2 = 210 g). Each 100 g has 0·2 g sodium, but as there are 210 g you will have to multiply by two and one-tenth (10 grams is one-tenth of 100 grams). Therefore, the sum will look like this: $0.2 \text{ g} \times 2.1 = 0.42$ g. However, that is the sodium content. To find the salt content, this figure will be multiplied by 2.5: $0.42 \text{ g} \times 2.5 = 1.05$ g.

Reflective activity

If Aurek does not manage to get this answer, would you feel comfortable explaining to him how to get the correct answer?

Over to you

Care management

If Aurek eats the portion of baked beans, how much salt will he be able to consume during the rest of the day if he follows the Department of Health's advice about limiting salt intake?

If Aurek has not eaten any salt that day and he then eats the portion of baked beans, he will need to restrict his salt intake to a maximum of 4.95 g over the rest of that day. The calculation would look like this: $6 - 1.05 \text{ g} = 4.95$ g.

Skills checklist

The number skills required in the previous calculations are division, multiplication and subtraction. If you have been unable to do this calculation or if you have had difficulty doing it, ask yourself:

- Did I understand what I was being asked to do?
- Did I have the number skills to carry out this calculation?
- Were there any number principles/formulae I could have used?

Perform the calculation. Ask yourself:

- Is it correct?
- How did I feel about the process?
- What do I need to do now?

Theory to practice

It is important that, as well as giving advice and information about healthy living, you check how much of this is understood by patients. This may involve checking patients' calculation skills.

RRRRRRRapid recap

Check your progress so far by working through each of the following points:

1. Provide an example of numeracy within this chapter that you may have to explain to the patient
2. Identify an example of calculation used in this patient's care
3. Explain how the calculation is relevant to this patient's care
4. Identify a source of help for those experiencing difficulties in some aspect of calculation.

References

BBC GCSE Bitesize Revision, www.bbc.co.uk/schools/gcsebitesize.

BBC Skillswise, www.bbc.co.uk/skillswise/tutors/expertcolumn/dyscalculia/index.shtml.

British Dyslexia Association, www.bdadyslexia.org.uk and www.bdadyslexia.org.uk/dyscalculia.html.

Department of Health (2000) *National Service Framework for Coronary Heart Disease*, Chapter 6, Heart Failure. Department of Health, London.

Food Standards Agency, www.food.gov.uk and www.salt.gov.uk.

Henderson, A. (1998) *Maths for the Dyslexic: a practical guide*. David Fulton, London.

Kearsley Bullen, R. (2003) *BBC KS3 Bitesize Revision*. BBC Worldwide, England.

Learn Direct, www.learndirect.org.uk and www.ufi.com/dyslexia/numeracy/implications.html.

Nigam, A., Bourassa, M., Fortier, A., Guertin, M.C. and Tardiff, J.C. (2006) The metabolic syndrome and its components and the long-term risk of death in patients with coronary heart disease. *American Heart Journal*, **152**(2), 514–521.

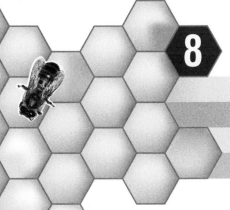

8

Exploring the nursing numeracy skills embedded in caring for a patient with a long-term condition:

Mr Mark Reynolds

Learning outcomes

By the end of this chapter you should be able to:

- Recognise where the numbers are in the nursing care of a patient with type 1 diabetes mellitus

- Calculate in a variety of nursing related contexts

- Use numeracy skills to explore the nursing care of this patient

- Identify sources of information relating to type 1 diabetes mellitus

Introduction

This chapter uses a case study to introduce you to some examples of numeracy when caring for a patient with type 1 diabetes mellitus.

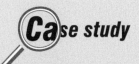

Case study

Mark Reynolds

Mark Reynolds is a 19-year-old physiotherapy student living in halls of residence. You are meeting him today, as his nurse specialist, to discuss how he is managing his diabetes. Mr Reynolds was diagnosed as having type 1 (insulin dependent) diabetes mellitus when he was six years old; this followed a brief period of hospitalisation when he developed chicken pox.

Mr Reynolds managed his diabetes successfully (under the watchful eye of his father) until he reached 14, when he started to take risks. He is more stable now, but is enjoying student life to the full, working and playing hard.

Mr Reynolds is following the recommended healthy diet for everyone, i.e. one that contains a balance of proteins, fats and carbohydrates. This is important for Mr Reynolds as he should be able to eat the same as his family and friends.

○━ Keywords

Glycaemic index

A way of describing
carbohydrates in terms of how
quickly they are absorbed into
the bloodstream

Theory to practice

When you work with patients like Mr Reynolds you need to be able to inform
them about healthy diets. People with type 1 diabetes mellitus are advised
to consider both what they eat and the timing of their meals (Vaughan
2005). It is important that the health professional involves the patient in
any discussion about their diabetes management, including diet. The diet
should enable the patient to maintain a normal weight, but it should also
be compatible with their lifestyle. Historically, people with diabetes focused
upon the carbohydrate content within their diet. However, it is important to
maintain the blood sugar (glycaemic) level, so it is now suggested that we
need to consider the **glycaemic index** (GI). Diabetes UK (www.diabetes.org.
uk) is a website for diabetics and it offers dietary advice including reducing
sugar and salt, eating complex carbohydrates, and eating lots of fruit and
vegetables. It is important that all health professionals give consistent advice,
so you might find a visit to this website worthwhile.

Over to you

Resource management

Diabetes mellitus is a common endocrine disorder (Avery 1998). The
Department of Health has a responsibility to review the health needs of
populations such as diabetics so that their needs are met in order to maintain
their health (see National Institute for Clinical Excellence at www.nice.org.uk).
Part of the information needed to undertake this health-needs analysis relates
to the number of diabetics in a given population, e.g. London.

Avery (1998) states that 'around 1·4 million people (3 per cent) in the UK'
have diabetes mellitus.

a. Express 1·4 million in numbers

b. If 1·4 million people equal 3% of the population of the UK, estimate the
population of the UK

c. Patients with type 1 diabetes mellitus make up approx 20% of the diabetic
population (Adam and Osborne 2005). How many people have type 1
diabetes mellitus? Express the answer in numbers.

a. One million, four hundred thousand is expressed in numbers as
1,400,000

b. To calculate the population of the UK, we need to find out what
1% equates to. As we know the number for 3% of the population,
we can do this by dividing 1,400,000 by 3. The calculation
is: 1,400,000 ÷ 3 = 466,667. In order to find the figure for
100% we then have to multiply this figure by 100. 466,667 ×
100 = 46,666,667. Remember, the answer should be stated in
units, so based on these figures, the population of the UK will

be approximately forty-six million, six hundred and sixty-six thousand, six hundred and sixty seven, which, expressed in numerals is 46,666,667

c. To calculate the number of people with type 1 diabetes mellitus, we know that the entire population of people with diabetes mellitus is 1·4 million (= 100%). We need to divide the number (1·4 million) by 100 to establish what 1% equates to, then multiply by 20, or multiply 1,400,000 by 20%, to find out the number of people with type 1 diabetes mellitus, thus:

$$\frac{1,400,\cancel{000}}{\cancel{100}} \times 20 = 14,000 \times 20 = 280,000$$

Or approximately two hundred and eighty thousand people will develop type 1 diabetes mellitus.

Skills checklist

The number skills required in this calculation are multiplication and division, using fractions, decimals and percentages. If you have been unable to do this calculation or if you have had difficulty with it, ask yourself:

● Did I understand what I was being asked to do?

● Did I have the number skills to carry out this calculation? If you are having difficulty understanding the problem, is it because you have literacy problems such as dyslexia? See the advice in Chapter 7, p. 116 relating to dyslexia about where to look for help

● Were there any number principles/formulae I could have used?

Perform the calculation. Ask yourself:

● Is it correct?

● How did I feel about the process?

● What do I need to do now?

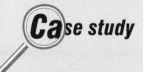

Case study

Case study continued

Mr Reynolds is on a mixture of short- and intermediate-acting insulin. He takes the intermediate-acting insulin morning and night, and during the day he uses an insulin pen containing short-acting insulin, giving himself a dose of insulin prior to meals. He relates this dose to his diet, estimating how many portions of carbohydrate he is about to consume. He also tests his blood glucose levels on a regular basis using blood glucose monitoring (BM) sticks. For every portion of carbohydrate he administers one unit of insulin. Therefore, for three portions of carbohydrate he will administer three units of insulin.

Theory to practice

When you work with patients like this you need to be able to educate them about their insulin. Insulin is a hormone produced by the pancreas. Diabetics need to inject themselves regularly with insulin in order to maintain normal blood sugar levels.

It is recommended that rapid-acting insulin be administered with each meal (Atkinson and Eisenbarth 2001) via pen or pump. This allows patients to react to blood glucose levels and therefore to deliver a pattern of insulin similar to the non-diabetic person. This is a very individualised way of managing care. The current trend is towards a combination of delivery method: syringe and pen, and several injections per day (NovoCare News 2000).

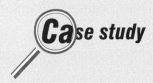

Case study continued

Mr Reynolds attends his appointment and confides that he has had some high BM readings lately. Although Mr Reynolds coped with his diabetes while living at home, he has had some problems since starting university. He does not have regular hours at university and finds the canteen food stodgy and high in carbohydrate. He has made some good friends, but their social life seems to consist mainly of nights in the student bar. As well as this, his university terms involve six weeks' theory in university and six weeks' placement, his most recent being in a stroke rehabilitation unit. He is finding his new lifestyle difficult to manage, and is missing the support from his father.

Mr Reynolds started his placement three weeks ago, but today he has had to get one of his friends to ring in sick for him. He has developed flu-like symptoms over the past two days, he cannot be bothered to cook any meals, and is now feeling decidedly unwell. He is feeling sick and has not eaten. Because of this he has decided not to take any insulin.

 Keywords

Hyperglycaemia
Raised blood sugar level
Glycosuria
Presence of glucose in the urine
Ketonuria
Presence of ketones in the urine

Theory to practice

You need to be able explain the problems associated with omitting insulin. Diabetes UK have some advice on their website that you could direct Mr Reynolds to (www.diabetes.org.uk).

Lack of insulin can result in the altered metabolism of proteins, fats and carbohydrates, which in turn results in **hyperglycaemia**, **glycosuria**, **ketonuria**, dehydration and electrolyte imbalance. There is a specific type of respiration associated with this condition, which occurs as a result of the acidosis which may accompany hyperglycaemia – kussmaul respirations (deep, laboured and sometimes sighing respirations).

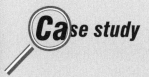

Case study

Case study continued
Over the past 48 hours Mr Reynolds has become increasingly lethargic and dehydrated. He is still complaining of nausea but also has abdominal pain, and his conscious level is deteriorating.

When his friends return to their accommodation, they are so concerned they call for an ambulance and he is admitted to a medical admissions unit. He is diagnosed as having diabetic ketoacidosis.

On admission to the unit, Mr Reynolds was suffering from hyperglycaemia, ketoacidosis and dehydration.

Theory to practice

You need to know current guidelines for the management of ketoacidosis. The *National Service Framework* (NSF) *for Diabetes* (Department of Health 2001) suggests that it is avoidable but potentially life threatening. Standard 7 of the NSF relates to the treatment and management of diabetic ketoacidosis.

Diabetic ketoacidosis (DKA) is an acute complication of type 1 diabetes mellitus and constitutes a medical emergency. It requires medical intervention and monitoring.

The treatment of diabetic ketoacidosis is determined by the individual patient's state, i.e. the patient's condition and what the laboratory tests reveal (Adam and Osborne 2005). NHS Trusts will have guidelines/protocols for dealing with this medical emergency, but according to Moore (2004) the aims of treatment will be to:

- Correct dehydration
- Reduce hyperglycaemia
- Correct acidosis.

Theory to practice

Diagnosis is confirmed by comprehensive assessment which would include testing for glycosuria and ketonuria, and observations of blood pressure, pulse and respirations.

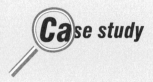

Case study continued

Blood and urine tests for the presence of glucose confirm that Mr Reynolds is hyperglycaemic; in view of his ketonuria, arterial blood is taken for blood gas analysis to assess the presence of metabolic ketoacidosis. This is confirmed; his pH is 7·12 (lower than normal) and his bicarbonate is 14 mmol/litre. His blood glucose level is 25 mmol/litre.

His blood pressure is 90/55 mmHg, pulse 140 bpm, respirations 30/minute and oxygen saturation is 85%.

Theory to practice

There are key nursing interventions to consider when caring for Mr Reynolds. He will need to be observed and monitored closely, i.e. an ECG to observe for arrhythmias, and central venous pressure (CVP), respiratory rate and pattern, blood pressure, pulse, blood gases, urinalysis and fluid balance should be checked. As his level of consciousness is deteriorating, it is important that his airway is maintained (Adam and Osborne 2005).

Correcting dehydration

To correct Mr Reynolds' dehydration, initially he is prescribed sodium chloride 0·9%. He requires large volumes administered rapidly.

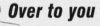 **Over to you**

Care management

Mr Reynolds is prescribed 2 litres of sodium chloride to be given in two hours, which is followed by 6 litres over eight hours, related to his ongoing blood tests and CVP measurements and ongoing monitoring of his blood glucose. This fluid is to be given by a gravity flow administration set.

Calculate the drip rate for the first two hours and the following eight hours.

To calculate the drip rate for 2 litres to be given in two hours, use the following formula:

$$\text{rate} = \frac{\text{volume (in ml)} \times \text{drop factor}}{\text{time (in hours)} \times \text{minutes in a hour}}$$

We will need to convert the litres into ml (1 litre = 1,000 ml) and consult the manufacturer's instructions on the wrapper of the giving set to establish the drop factor (this is often 20 drops per ml for clear fluids).

$$\text{rate} = \frac{2\!\!\!^1,000 \times 2\theta}{2\!\!\!^1 \times 6\theta}$$

Remember: although these are easy numbers we can still 'cancel out' by using common denominators.

$$\text{rate} = \frac{2,000}{6} = 333.3 = 334 \text{ drops per minute}$$

To calculate the drip rate for 6 litres over eight hours use the following formula:

$$\text{rate} = \frac{\text{volume (in ml)} \times \text{drops per ml}}{\text{time (in hours)} \times \text{minutes in a hour}}$$

$$\text{rate} = \frac{6\!\!\!^1,000 \times 2\theta}{8 \times 6\!\!\!^1\theta} = \frac{2,000}{8} = 250 \text{ drops per minute}$$

These drip rates may seem unmanageable, but we are trying to correct his dehydration by giving fluid quickly. This is a life-threatening condition. We would use a mechanical/electronic device such as a volumetric pump as we would be unable to count this drip rate.

Reducing hyperglycaemia

Mr Reynolds will need to receive an intravenous infusion of insulin to reduce his raised blood sugar levels. Correcting his dehydration will have helped to reduce his blood glucose, but he will need to receive a short-acting insulin and the insulin is usually given intravenously in order to act quickly. This is usually administered as an infusion of 50 units of soluble insulin in 50 ml sodium chloride 0·9%.

This is normally delivered by a syringe driver (infusion pump) at the rate of 1 unit per ml. Lewis (2000) recommends a reduction in his blood glucose of approximately 5 mmol/hour.

Adam and Osborne (2005) recommend that a low rate infusion of 2–5 units/hour should be commenced, but that this should be monitored carefully in relation to the patient's ongoing blood glucose levels, which would be measured hourly. When his blood glucose returns to normal, his urine is free from ketones and he is eating again he can resume his insulin via the subcutaneous route.

> ## Over to you
>
> **Care management**
> If the prescription is for 5 units per hour, what would the delivery rate be?

Using a medical device such as a syringe driver, which is based upon the delivery of ml of fluid per hour, the following formula would be used to calculate the delivery of intravenous fluids:

$$\text{delivery rate (ml per hour)} = \frac{\text{volume (in ml)}}{\text{time (in hours)}}$$

$$\text{delivery rate} = \frac{5 \; (5 \text{ units} = 5 \text{ ml})}{1} = 5 \text{ ml/hour}$$

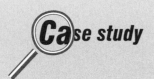

Case study continued
Mr Reynolds' blood glucose has now dropped to 12 mmol/litre. His prescription is therefore changed to 2 units per hour and he has commenced intravenous glucose.

Calculate the delivery rate for this prescription.

$$\text{delivery rate} = \frac{2}{1} = 2 \text{ ml/hour}$$

Skills checklist

The number skills required in this calculation are multiplication and division. If you have been unable to do this or if you have had difficulty doing it, ask yourself:

- Did I understand what I was being asked to do?
- Were there any number principles/formulae I could have used?

There are two formulae we can use when calculating intravenous fluid delivery according to whether we are using a gravity flow administration set and a syringe driver.

Perform the calculation. Ask yourself:

- Is it correct?
- How did I feel about the process?
- What do I need to do now?

Key points / Top tips

- The numbers referring to the 'strength' of the sodium chloride do not need to be considered for this equation
- Cancelling out numbers makes the numerals more manageable, but you can decide how far you want to take this process
- When cancelling numbers remember you must carry out the same action both on the top and bottom.

Over to you

Care management

Adam and Osborne (2005) suggest that when the patient's blood sugar has dropped to 10 mmol/litre, then glucose should be added to the prescription for intravenous fluid replacement. They recommend 100 ml/hour

Calculate the infusion rate for Mr Reynolds' glucose if the prescription is for 5% glucose 100 ml/hour.

You need to use the following formula:

$$\text{rate} = \frac{\text{volume (in ml)} \times \text{drop factor}}{\text{time (in hours)} \times \text{minutes in a hour}}$$

We have used this calculation earlier in this chapter, so you should be familiar with the process. These are very straightforward numbers, so you may decide not to cancel them.

$$\text{rate} = \frac{1,000 \times 20}{1 \times 60} = \frac{2,000}{60} = 33 \cdot 3 \text{ dpm} = 34 \text{ dpm}$$

Correcting acidosis

Theory to practice

Metabolic acidosis is characterised by an increase in total body acid which causes an imbalance in the pH level.

Intravenous sodium bicarbonate will be considered in ketoacidosis, but its role is controversial as it has the potential to cause alkalosis and hypocalcaemia (Moore 2004). However, this would not be indicated for Mr Reynolds as his blood pH is over 7·1.

RRRRR**Rapid recap**

Check your progress so far by working through each of the following points:

1. Provide an example of numeracy within this chapter which you might need to explain to the patient

2. Identify an example of calculation used in this patient's care

3. Explain how the calculation is relevant to this patient's care

4. Identify a source of help for those experiencing difficulties in some aspect of calculation

If you have difficulty with more than one of these questions, read through the section again to refresh your understanding before moving on.

References

Adam, S.K. and Osborne, S. (2005) *Critical Care Nursing. Science and Practice*, 2nd edn. Oxford University Press, Oxford.

Atkinson, M.A. and Eisenbarth, G.S. (2001) Type 1 diabetes: New perspectives on disease pathogenesis an treatment. *The Lancet*, **358**(9277), 221–230.

Avery, L. (1998) Diabetes mellitus types 1 and 2: an overview. *Nursing Standard*, **13**(8), 35–38.

Diabetes UK, www.diabetes.org.uk.

Department of Health (2001) *National Service Framework for Diabetes*. Department of Health, London.

Lewis, R. (2000) Diabetic emergencies: Part 2. Hyperglycaemia. *Accident and Emergency Nursing*. **8**, 24–30.

Moore, T. (2004) Diabetic emergencies in adults. *Nursing Standard*, **18**(46), 45–52.

National Institute for Health and Clinical Excellence, www.nice.org.uk.

NovoCare News (2000) Novofine: very fine needles indeed. Ideal length for needles. *Diabetes Today*, **4**(3), 2.

Vaughan, L. (2005) Dietary guidelines for the management of diabetes. *Nursing Standard*, **19**(44), 56–64.

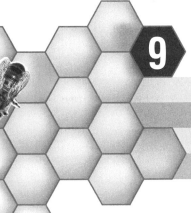

9 Exploring the nursing numeracy skills embedded in caring for a patient in an acute care setting:

Mrs Gina Lloyd

Learning outcomes

By the end of this chapter you should be able to:

- Recognise where numbers are in the nursing care of patients such as Mrs Gina Lloyd
- Calculate in a variety of nursing-related contexts
- Use numeracy skills to explore the nursing care of Mrs Gina Lloyd

Introduction

In order to explore some of the numeracy skills embedded in caring for patients in an acute care setting, this chapter introduces you to Mrs Gina Lloyd.

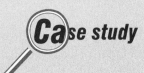

Case study

Gina Lloyd

Mrs Gina Lloyd, 38, has been admitted this morning for a laparoscopic cholecystectomy (non-invasive removal of the gall bladder) following frequent bouts of severe pain in her upper right abdominal quadrant accompanied by nausea and vomiting. Following a diagnosis of cholelithiasis (gallstones), Mrs Lloyd followed a low-fat diet, although she felt it did not make any difference to the frequency or severity of her symptoms. As a result, she has lost 1·2 kg, and at her pre-admission assessment she was noted as weighing 67·27 kg. Her vital signs were recorded as BP 125/75mmHg, pulse 82bpm and regular. Accompanying Mrs Lloyd was her husband Gerald, who, after seeing her settled into the ward, went to work. He is taking holiday from tomorrow for two weeks in order to take Gina home and look after her and their eight-year-old daughter Ami. Initially, Gina appears to make an uneventful post-operative recovery, her vital signs are all within normal limits, there is no leakage from her wound sites and she is pain free. After about an hour she begins to complain of generalised abdominal pain, which she says is not as severe as some of the episodes of pain that she had before her surgery. There is no change in any of her vital signs and no leakage from her wounds. Gina then begins to complain of severe abdominal pain that has become more localised to the right epigastrium. Her vital signs are BP 120/75mmHg, pulse rate 88bpm and regular, respiration rate 19, O_2 sats 98% and temperature 37°C. Over the next hour she becomes increasingly restless. Her vital signs begin to change: BP is now 95/60mmHg, P 118bpm, R 18, O_2 sats 89%, her skin looks pale and moist. Over the following hour her vital signs (measured by Dinamap) are as follows:

Time	BP	Pulse	Resps	Temp
14.30	90/60	122 regular	18	37
14.45	85/60	125 regular	24	37
15.00	90/60	128 regular, thready	20	37
15.15	80/55	130 regular, thready	20	37·2
15.30	80/55	134 regular, thready	22	37·2

Over to you

Care management

Using Gina's vital signs given above and the Modified Early Warning Score (MEWS) chart shown in Table 9.1, identify Gina's MEWS score for each of her vital signs at the times they were recorded

14.30 =

14.45 =

15.00 =

15.15 =

15.30 =

Table 9.1 Modified Early Warning Score

Score	3	2	1	0	1	2	3
Systolic blood pressure (mmHg)	<70	71–80	81–100	101–199		>200	
Heart rate (bpm)		<40	41–50	51–100	101–110	111–129	>130
Respiratory rate (bpm)		<9		9–14	15–20	21–29	>30
Temperature (°C)		<35		35–38·4		>38·5	
AVPU score				**Alert**	Reacting to Voice	Reacting to Pain	**Unresponsive**

*Source: Subbe, C.P., Kruger, M., Rutherford, P. and Gemmel, L. (2001) Validation of modified early warning score in medical admissions. Quality Journal of Medicine, **94**, 521–526, by permission of Oxford University Press.*

Gina's MEWS would look like this:

14.30 Systolic BP 1, Heart rate 2, Resp rate 1 = 4

14.45 Systolic BP 1, Heart rate 2, Resp rate 2 = 5

15.00 Systolic BP 1, Heart rate 2, Resp rate 1 = 4

15.15 Systolic BP 2, Heart rate 3, Resp rate 1 = 6

15.30 Systolic BP 2, Heart rate 3, Resp rate 1 = 6

Skills checklist

The number skill asked for in this calculation is addition. You also need to be able to read from a chart and interpret data. If you have been unable to do this calculation or you have had difficulty, ask yourself:

- Did I understand what I was being asked to do?
- Did I have the number skills to carry out this calculation? If you are having difficulty understanding the problem, is it because you have literacy problems such as dyslexia? See the advice in Chapter 7 (p. 116 relating to dyslexia) about where to look for help
- Were there any number principles/formulae you could have used?

Perform the calculation. Ask yourself:

- Is it correct?
- How did you feel about the process?
- What do you need to do now?

Theory to practice

It is important that you understand how physiological data reflects the patient's condition and how the observations you make of the patient's vital signs, behaviour and condition can combine to indicate either deterioration or improvement. This will help you to recognise changes in the patient's condition and refer them appropriately for medical intervention. Numerical recognition and interpretation is fundamental to this understanding. One method which is becoming more commonly used to help staff make such interpretations is the Modified Early Warning Score (MEWS). This is where 'each vital sign is allocated a score and the score increases or decreases in relation to the patient's condition. The higher the score the greater the risk of the patient's condition deteriorating' (Department of Health 2000). A raised MEWS reflects a patient's risk of increased mortality. Scores of five and over indicate that the patient's condition is giving concern and requires immediate resuscitation measures (Morgan *et al.* 1997; Subbe *et al.* 2001).

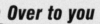**Reflective activity**

Gina's MEWS indicates her deteriorating condition. Consider what actions you would take in a similar situation. If you are not sure that you have this knowledge and understanding, consider highlighting this for your professional development in your Professional Portfolio.

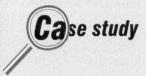

Case study continued

Following an examination by the surgeon, Gina returns to theatre for an exploratory laparotomy. Staff Nurse Baxter is the scrub nurse managing Gina's surgery. Once Gina's abdomen is opened it quickly becomes evident that Gina is bleeding into her abdomen, and on further exploration it becomes apparent that she is bleeding from liver lacerations. Towards the end of this surgery, before the surgeon begins to close the abdomen, Staff Nurse Baxter begins to account for the instruments and mops/swabs used during the operation. The fluid that Gina has lost into her abdomen, which has been aspirated into the suction jar, also has to be accounted for so that Gina's cumulative blood loss can be assessed. Staff Nurse Baxter has counted out 17 bundles of large (15 g dry weight) raytec gauzes (packs) and eight bundles of small (10 g dry weight) raytec gauzes (mops).

Over to you

Risk management

As there are five (15 g) packs in a bundle and five (10 g) mops in a bundle, how many individual packs and mops has Staff Nurse Baxter made available to the surgical team?

Well done if you said that 85 (15 g) packs and 40 (10 g) mops were made available for the surgical team. If you did not get this answer, recheck your calculations and, if you are using a calculator, check each of your data entries carefully. The calculation for the pack/mop total will be the number of bundles multiplied by the number of raytec gauzes that are in each bundle (always five), i.e. $17 \times 5 = 85$. If you did not get this answer, can you see what the problem is? The problem here is that the total number of raytec gauzes will always be a larger number than the number of bundles opened. So, in order to get a larger number you have to multiply the two totals (number of bundles × number of raytec gauzes in a bundle).

One way of calculating this would be to break up the sum into two parts: first $5 \times 10 = 50$, then, $5 \times 7 = 35$. After this, add the two totals together: $50 + 35 = 85$. Therefore, there are 85 (15 g) packs.

The calculation for the total mops will be $5 \times 8 = 40$. Again, you could do the sum as mental arithmetic or you could use a calculator. Therefore, there are 40 (10 g) mops.

Skills checklist

The number skills required in this calculation are multiplication and addition. If you have been unable to do this calculation or you have had difficulty, ask yourself:

- Did I understand what I was being asked to do?
- Did I have the number skills to carry out this calculation?
- Were there any number principles/formulae I could have used?

Perform the calculation. Ask yourself:

- Is it correct?
- How did I feel about the process?

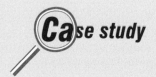

Case study

Case study continued

In reality, each wet raytec gauze would be weighed. Here each 1 g of raytec gauze (pack or mop) weighs approximately 1 g when it is dry and each 1 g dry weight has the ability to absorb approximately 1 ml of blood.

Over to you

Risk management

How much blood will a) each pack (15 g dry weight) and b) each mop (10 g dry weight) have the capacity to absorb?

Congratulations if you said that a) each pack (15 g dry weight) would absorb approximately 15 ml and b) each mop (10 g dry weight) has the capacity to absorb 10 ml.

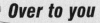

Over to you

Risk management

So, if each pack (15 g dry weight) is able to absorb approximately 15 ml and each mop (10 g dry weight) has the capacity to absorb approximately 10 ml, how much will each of the packs and mops weigh when fully saturated with blood?

Nice work if you found the answer to be each pack (15 g dry weight) would weigh 30 g (15 g dry material + 15 ml blood, equivalent to 15 g weight = 30 g). Consequently, each mop (10 g dry weight) would weigh 20 g (10 g + 10 ml/g = 20 g). Although this approximation is reasonably accurate, bear in mind that not all raytec gauzes will all absorb the same amount of fluid.

So, 71 (15 g) blood-soaked packs and 10 (10 g) blood-soaked mops have been accounted for. In the suction jar there is 1,791 ml of blood-stained fluid. In order to help estimate Gina's blood loss, Staff Nurse Baxter will have to count the fluid loss contained in the raytec gauzes as well as the fluid caught in the suction jar.

Over to you

Care management

How much blood will there be in total in the used packs (15 g) and the blood-soaked mops (10 g)?

There are 71 packs and 10 mops used and discarded, so the total blood loss absorbed by the packs and mops is (71 × 15 ml) + (10 × 10 ml) = 1,065 ml + 100 ml = 1,165 ml. So the blood loss absorbed by the packs and mops is 1,165 ml.

Over to you

Care management

Near the end of the operation Staff Nurse Baxter has to estimate the blood loss. How much blood will Gina have lost?

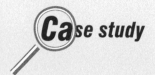

Case study

Case study continued

Gina has lost approximately 2,956 ml of blood. If you did not get this answer, did you remember to add in the blood loss collected by suctioning? Total blood loss will be the sum of all the blood loss, and this will be estimated by adding the amount from the mops (1,165 ml) to the amount in the suction jar (1,791 ml). This calculation will look like this: 1,165 ml + 1,791 ml = 2,956 ml. To check that this answer is correct, you can work the calculation backwards, so, 2,956 ml – 1,791 ml (the amount in the suction jar) = 1,165 ml. This is the total from the blood-soaked mops, so the answer is correct.

Key points | **Top tips**

- There may be more than one right way to calculate the answer, but whichever way you use, you must ensure that you have the correct answer

- If you cannot remember formulae or how to work something out, take Pólya's advice (Pólya 1990) and assess, plan, implement and evaluate (see Chapter 3, p. 42)

- If you feel yourself becoming anxious/using negative coping strategies, remember you can overcome this (see Chapter 2, p. 29)

- If you use a calculator, be aware of calculator data entry errors. Establish a habit of checking every entry that you make

- Estimate the answer first so that you have a rough idea of what the answer should be

- Working the calculation backwards is one way of checking if the answer is correct.

Over to you

Risk management

How many unused packs and mops should there be at Gina's operation site? Use Table 9.2 to help you with your calculation.

There should be 14 packs (15 g) and 30 mops (10 g) left at the operation site. 85 packs (15 g) and 40 mops (10 g) were made available to the surgical team, and 71 packs and 10 mops have been used and discarded. So, as there will be fewer left at the operation site than at the beginning of surgery, the calculation will be subtraction and it will look like this: 85 – 71 = 14; 40 – 10 = 30.

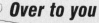

Over to you

Risk management

Complete the count board in Table 9.2 using the information given above and calculate the running totals in each of the relevant columns

See Appendix E for the completed count board. Check yours against that one.

Table 9.2 Count board blood loss

Packs (15 g)			Mops (10 g)		
Number of packs	**Running total**	**Blood loss (ml) running total**	**Number of mops**	**Running total**	**Blood loss (ml) running total**
6			4		
5			2		
3			3		
7			1		
2					
4					
5					
3					
7					
9					
4					
6					
7					
3					

Theory to practice

In this case study, you will need to understand your responsibilities as the scrub nurse in relation to patient and staff safety. In this scenario and in relation to the calculations required these responsibilities are threefold:

1. You need to be aware of how many raytec gauzes are available
2. You should know how many raytec gauzes have been used
3. You should know much fluid has been lost at the operation site so that this can be replaced.

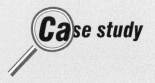
Case study

Case study continued
It is Gina's second post-op day. She appears to be recovering well. Earlier in the day Gina's blood transfusion was replaced with an intravenous infusion. It is 1 p.m. and the infusate needs to be replaced. Gina has been prescribed 500 ml of 0.9% sodium chloride over four hours.

> ### Over to you
>
> **Risk management**
> You have to put up Gina's next bag of infusate. What flow rate should you key into the IV controller? (The volumetric pump that you will use works by measuring flow rate in ml/hr.)

You would key in 125 ml per hour. Your calculation should look like this:

$$\frac{500 \text{ ml}}{4 \text{ hrs}} = 125 \text{ ml/hr}$$

In this example, you need to find out how many ml have to be infused every hour. In this instance you know two things:

1. Volume to be infused (0.5 litre or 500 ml)
2. Infusion duration, i.e. the length of time that the infusion is expected to run (four hours).

If you did not get the correct answer the following explanation will clarify how to solve this particular problem.

You are asked to find out the rate in ml/hour. You know that the infusion is to run for four hours and that the total volume of the infusion is 500 ml, so you need to find out how many 4s there are in 500 ml. This means dividing 500 by 4. The calculation will look like this:

$$\frac{500}{4}$$

As the amount of fluid infused per hour will be a much smaller amount than the whole amount of the infusion, you will have to divide the whole amount by the length of time that the infusion is expected to run (duration), i.e. divide the volume (500 ml) by the duration of the infusion in hours (4). The calculation will look like this:

$$\frac{500}{4}$$

This will give you the ml/hr.

Skills checklist

The number skill required in this calculation is division. If you have been unable to do this calculation or you have had difficulty, ask yourself:

- Did I understand what I was being asked to do?
- Did I have the number skills to carry out this calculation?
- Were there any number principles/formulae I could have used?

Perform the calculation. Ask yourself:

- Is it correct?
- How did I feel about the process?
- What do I need to do now?

Key points Top tips

- If you use infusion devices in the area in which you work, you should know how to use them
- In the interest of patient safety and to fulfil your NMC Code of Conduct (2002) obligations, you should have attended the Trust's training programme.

Theory to practice

There is a standard formula for working out intravenous infusion rates for either manually controlled IV administration or electronically controlled delivery. The standard formula is:

$$\text{rate (drops per minute)} = \frac{\text{volume (ml)} \times \text{drop factor}}{\text{time (in hours)} \times 60}$$

Remember that the drop factor varies with the giving set used. The drop factor is the number of drops per ml that the giving set delivers. As a general rule, microdrip tubing, or paediatric tubing as it is sometimes called, universally delivers 60 drops per ml. It is used when either very small or very precise volumes are to be infused. Consequently, microdrip tubing is used when giving IV fluids to children or sometimes in adult nursing when more exact control is required but an electronic device is unavailable. This contrasts with macrodrip tubing, used most commonly in adult nursing, which varies depending on whether the giving set is being used to transfuse blood or infuse clear fluids. Commonly, blood-giving sets have a drop factor of 15 drops per ml, while IV-giving sets for administering clear fluids have a drop factor of 20 drops per ml. (NB: Different manufacturers also use different drop factors in their tubing, so make sure that you check the packaging for the information.)

Over to you

Risk management

Gina was prescribed 1 litre of 5% dextrose prescribed to run for eight hours. The drop factor is 20 drops per ml. If you were using a gravity flow IV infusion, how many drops per minute would this be?

Congratulations if you answered 42. If you worked out the answer using a calculator you will have got 41·66. . . . Normally, that calculation would be rounded up to 42. If you did not get this answer, recheck your calculations. It could be that you have misused your calculator. If your calculations are still not right, check the information about using calculators (see Appendix G).

In this situation you have to find out two things:

1. How many drops are in the bag of fluid
2. How many minutes the infusion will run.

Using the formula identified in Theory to practice earlier, your calculation will look like this:

$$\frac{1,000}{8} \times \frac{20}{60} = \frac{20,000}{480} = 41\cdot66 \ldots$$

(NB: For further clarification, see Chapter 4, p. 78.)

Over to you

Risk management

Figure 9.1 shows Gina's fluid balance chart for her second post-op day. Total up the chart. Is Gina in positive or negative fluid balance?

FLUID BALANCE CHART

Name   ...Gina Lloyd...................... Hospital Number ...123zz45................. **Date** ......1.9.06......

| | | | INTAKE | | | | | OUTPUT | | | |
Time	IV Line 1 Flagyl	IV Line 2 Cefuroxime	IV Line 3	Oral	Running Total		Drain 1	Drain 2	Urine	Running Total
			Packed Cells							
0800	110	100	125				150	125	32	
0900			125				130	120	36	
1000			125				132	120	36	
1100			125				130	120	40	
1200			0.9%Sodium Chloride 125				130	115	41	
1300			125				130	115	45	
1400			125				126	115	45	
1500			125				46	68	45	
1600	110	100	125				24	48	45	
1700			5% Glucose 125	30			20	24	45	
1800			125	30					50	
1900			125	30			10	5	50	
2000			125	30					45	
2100			125	60					40	
2200			125	60					40	
2300			125						38	
2400	110	100	125						42	
0100			125	60					44	
0200									40	
0300			Hartmann's Solution 125						58	
0400			125						65	
0500			125						62	
0600			125						68	
0700			125						60	
Totals										

Insensible loss 500

TOTAL INTAKE: **TOTAL OUTPUT:**

BALANCE:

Figure 9.1 *Fluid balance chart*

Key points **Top tips**

- Addition can be done in a number of different ways. You can add the numbers together as they are or recognise the nearest whole number for each of the numbers, add these together, then subtract the differences between the number to be added and the whole number, e.g. when adding 59, 37, 25 and 68 you could add 60, 40, 30 and 70, making 200. You would then subtract the total of 1, 3, 5 and 2, which is 11; 200 − 11 = 189

- You can use a series of sums or add them together in one go. For example, 13 + 12 + 56 + 534 + 793 + 63 + 95 + 664 + 434 + 29 + 7 + 18 could be added together in two groups, i.e. 13 + 12 + 56 + 63 + 95 + 29 + 7 + 18 = 293; 534 + 793 + 664 + 434 = 2,425. Then the sum of the two groups added together: 293 + 2,425 = 2,718

- You can write the numbers down rather than rely on mental arithmetic.

Theory to practice

Gina's fluid chart shows a positive fluid balance, suggesting that she may be retaining fluid. However, consideration must be given to recognising her previous and ongoing fluid loss. In situations such as this you need to have the knowledge and skills to assess accurately how well the patient is hydrated, as well as assessing their circulatory volume. Assessing the circulatory volume and state of hydration in patients such as Gina means evaluating more than their fluid balance records. Assessment also involves collating the following information: serum electrolyte measurements, examination of the patient's skin and tongue, and their mental state. Analysis of this information will enable you to identify signs and symptoms of dehydration or fluid overload. If you are not sure how to do this, you should identify this in your portfolio and work towards developing your knowledge and skills in this area.

Compare your completed fluid balance chart with the one in Appendix F.

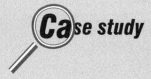 **Case study**

Case study continued
In order to prevent Gina becoming malnourished, she has been seen by the dietitian and is now having Total Parenteral Nutrition. Apart from IV glucose, she is prescribed 500 ml of Intralipid 20% every 24 hours.

> ## Over to you
>
> **Care management**
> Intralipid will give Gina 8,400 kJ/litre (www.bnf.org). As many of us are more familiar with energy requirements expressed in kilocalories than kilojoules, converting the kilojoules to kilocalories may help you to understand more fully whether Gina's metabolic demands are being met. How many kilocalories will the Intralipid give her over a 24-hour period? (NB: 1,000 kJ = 238·8 kcalories).

Well done if you worked out that the answer is 1,003 kcal. If you did not get this answer, re-enter your calculations into your calculator and check each data entry carefully, or check your workings-out. We know that there are 8,400 kJ in 1 litre of Intralipid and that Gina has been prescribed 500 ml or half a litre of Intralipid every 24 hours. So, there will be 8·4 times more kcalories than kilojoules in every litre. There are two ways to work this out:

1. In a litre 238·8 × 8·4 = 2,005·92 (or rounded up = 2,006). However, Gina is having 500 ml (half as much), so this would have to be divided by 2 = 1,002·96 (or rounded up = 1,003). The equation would therefore be written like this:

$$\frac{238\cdot8}{2} \times 8\cdot4 \ = \ 1{,}002\cdot96 \text{ or rounded up} = 1{,}003$$

2. In 500 ml of Intralipid there will be 4,200 kilojoules ($^{8{,}400}/_2$ = 4,200). 238·8 × 4·2 = 1,002·96 kilocalories or rounded up = 1,003. This calculation would be written in an equation like this:

$$\frac{8{,}400}{2} \times 238\cdot8 \ = \ 1{,}002\cdot96 \text{ or rounded up} = 1{,}003$$

Skills checklist

The number skills required in this calculation are division and multiplication as well as rounding up and down. If you have been unable to do this calculation or you have had difficulty, ask yourself:

● Did I understand what I was being asked to do?

● Did I have the number skills to carry out this calculation?

● Were there any number principles/formulae I could have used?

Perform the calculation. Ask yourself:

● Is it correct?

● How did I feel about the process?

● What do I need to do now?

Theory to practice

So that you can put your numeracy skills into perspective in care situations such as this, you need to understand:

● Why your patient needs to have parenteral or enteral nutrition

● Which route the evidence suggests should be the preferred route

● Which would be suitable feeds to use

● What nutritional intake would be necessary to meet the needs of the patient being cared for.

Alongside this, you should understand the extra care that would have to be incorporated into the patient's care plan as a result of:

● Psychological and social implications for the patient

● The impact of malnutrition on the immune system

● The influence on the mouth of not eating or drinking.

(See www.bapen.org.uk)

Over to you

Risk management

Look at the information above. Given Gina's condition and the surgery she has had in the last few days, do you consider that this will be an adequate intake of nutrients for her?

Gina will be getting approximately half the number of kilocalories recommended for the average well woman. Gina's body will have had a great demand for energy resources in the last few days and she has not been taking any oral food. As a result, her body will be unable to meet her metabolic demands, so she will be becoming malnourished. However, while products like Intralipid have great advantages, they also have disadvantages (see www.bnf.org.uk) and consequently they need to be introduced over a few days.

Theory to practice – Care management

When working in areas where enteral and parenteral nutrition are used, you should have an understanding of the metabolic demands of disease and injury. You should also be able to assess patients' nutritional status. For patients such as Gina who cannot easily be weighed and measured, there are alternative means at your disposal that will help you to identify whether a patient is well nourished or not, e.g. the MUST assessment tool (British Association of Parenteral and Enteral Nutrition, available at www.bapen.org.uk).

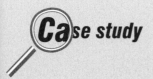

Case study continued

The surgical ward sister running the ward in which Gina is a patient feels that the skill mix needs to be reviewed given the changing needs of the patients who are now admitted to the ward. As part of this review she is exploring whether there are any financial resources available within the staffing budget. The ward has a monthly staffing budget of whole time equivalents (wtes), as shown in Table 9.3.

Table 9.3 Monthly staffing budget

Establishment	Band	Allocated budget (£)	Actual budget (£)
3 wtes	6	6,277	6,277
11 wtes	5	21,300	19,196
2 wtes	3	2,282	2,282
4 wtes	2	6,101	4,067
1 wtes	1	989	364

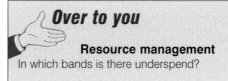

Over to you

Resource management

In which bands is there underspend?

From the information given in Table 9.3, you should have identified that there is an underspend in bands 5, 2 and 1. The table shows that the allocated and actual monthly budgets for bands 6 and 3 are the same, so there are no overspends or underspends in either of these bands. However, subtracting the actual monthly budget from the allocated monthly budget in bands 5, 2 and 1 demonstrates an underspend in each of these bands. Your calculations should look like this:

Band 5: £21,300 – £19,196 = £2,104

Band 2: £6,101 – £4,067 = £2,034

Band 1: £989 – £364 = £625

Remember, you can check your answer by working backwards, i.e. band 1: £625 + £364 = £989; band 2: £2,034 + £4,067 = £6,101; band 5: £2,104 + £19,196 = £21,300.

Theory to practice

The number skills required in this calculation are subtraction and, to check your answer, addition. If you have been unable to do this calculation or you have had difficulty, ask yourself:

● Did I understand what I was being asked to do?

● Did I have the number skills to carry out this calculation?

● Were there any number principles/formulae I could have used?

Perform the calculation. Ask yourself:

● Is it correct?

● How did I feel about the process?

● What do I need to do now?

Over to you

Resource management

Identify the monthly and yearly savings that could be made as a result of the underspend on salaries.

The underspend will give you a monthly saving of £4,763. Over a year this would amount to £57,156. The monthly savings will be the sum of the totals of bands 1, 2 and 5, so your calculation would look like this: £2,104 + £2,034 + £625 = £4,763. In order to find how much this would be over a year, the monthly savings would be multiplied by 12 (12 months in a year). The calculation would be written down like this: £4,763 × 12 = £57,156. To check that the answer is correct, you could work it backwards, i.e. £57,156 ÷ 12 = £4,763.

Theory to practice

In situations such as this you would have to consider what knowledge and skills the staff should have in order to meet the changing needs of the ward. The NHS Knowledge and Skills Framework (Agenda for Change Project Team 2004) would be a valuable resource for this. This information would then feed into the reconfiguration, perhaps giving new opportunities for staff development.

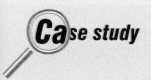 *Case study*

Case study continued

The ward's annual dressings budget is £3,800. The expenditure on dressings to date on the statement dated 30 September is £1,650.

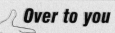 *Over to you*

Resource management

How much is left in the dressings budget for the rest of the year?

Well done if you said that there is £2,150 left in the dressings budget for the rest of the year. The calculation would be the annual budget minus the expenditure to date. So the equation would be £3,800 – £1,650 = £2,150. You can check your answer by working backwards: £2,150 + £1,650 = £3,800.

Skills checklist

The number skills required in this calculation are subtraction and addition (to check your answer). If you have been unable to do this calculation or you had difficulty, ask yourself:

● Did I understand what I was being asked to do?
● Did I have the number skills to carry out this calculation?
● Were there any number principles/formulae I could have used?

Perform the calculation. Ask yourself:

- Is it correct?
- How did I feel about the process?
- What do I need to do now?

The tissue viability link nurse would like to change the dressing used for discharging wounds to a dressing that is initially more expensive but requires changing less often. The extra cost of the dressings would amount to £35 per month. You agree to try this for three months and will find the savings from other areas of the budget if necessary.

Over to you

Resource management
What will be the total cost of the three-month trial of the new wound dressings?

Nice work if you calculated that the total costs for the three-month trial will be £930. If you did not get this answer, check your calculations again. First, you need to find what a month's budget is. You do this by dividing the expenditure to date by the number of months in the financial year to date, i.e. £1,650 ÷ 6 − £275. Then add the extra cost of the new dressings each month at £35, i.e. £275 + £35 = £310. As the extra costs will be for three months you need to multiply this answer by the number of months £310 × 3 = £930. The equation would look like this: $(1,650 \div 6 + 35) \times 3 = 930$.

Skills checklist

The number skills required in this calculation are division, addition and multiplication. If you have been unable to do this calculation or you have had difficulty, ask yourself:

- Did I understand what I was being asked to do?
- Did I have the number skills to carry out this calculation?
- Were there any number principles/formulae I could have used?

Perform the calculation. Ask yourself:

- Is it correct?
- How did I feel about the process?
- What do I need to do now?

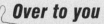

Over to you

Resource management
If the new dressings are successful and are to be used for the rest of the
financial year and, given that the monthly budget for dressings remains
unchanged, project how much the overspend will be.

Nice work if you spotted that the dressing budget will have an
underspend of £290 if the monthly amount spent on dressings
does not get any larger before the end if the financial year. If you
did not arrive at this answer, did you remember that the
financial year runs from the 1 April to 31 March? So,
remembering that the statement date was 30 September, the
budget has another six months to run. You can calculate this in
two ways:

1. In the first six months of the year £1,650 has been spent on
    dressings, leaving £2,150 for the second six months. So, if
    the cost of dressings does not rise in this time the projected
    underspend will be £290. During the next six months it is
    predicted that £1,860 will be spent on dressings. Subtract this
    total from the amount left in the budget (£2,150), which
    leaves an underspend of £290. The calculation will look like
    this: £2,150 – £1,860 = £290.

2. Alternatively, you can use the monthly spend on the budget to
    date × the number of months the budget still has left to run
    (£275 × 6 = £1,650). The extra cost of dressings at £35 for
    six months will be £210 (£35 × 6 = £210). These two totals
    are then added together, which equals £1,860. The calculation
    will look like this: £1,650 + £210 = £1,860. This total
    (£1,860) is then added to the budget spend to date to give
    you a projected year's total of £3,510 (£1,860 + £1,650 =
    £3,510). This total is subtracted from the annual budget of
    £3,800 (£3,800 – £3,510 = £290), which equates to a
    projected underspend of £290.

This underspend could then be **vired** to meet the costs of
other things (although it will not buy many staff hours), or it
may be more prudent for it to be kept in hand for a few months
in case unforeseen increases in the dressings budget arise later
in the financial year.

⚷ *Keywords*

Vired
NHS financial jargon for
transferring money from one
account to another one

Skills checklist

The number skills required in this calculation are addition, subtraction and multiplication. If you have been unable to do this calculation or you have had difficulty, ask yourself:

- Did I understand what I was being asked to do?
- Did I have the number skills to carry out this calculation?
- Were there any number principles/formulae I could have used?

Perform the calculation. Ask yourself:

- Is it correct?
- How did I feel about the process?
- What do I need to do now?

Rapid recap

Check your progress so far by working through each of the following points:

1. Provide an example of numeracy within this chapter that you may have to explain to a student nurse
2. Explain how this calculation would be relevant to a student nurse
3. Identify a source of help for those experiencing difficulties in some aspect of the calculation

If you have difficulty with one of these questions, read through the section again to refresh your understanding before moving on.

References

British Association for Parenteral and Enteral Nutrition, www.bapen.org.uk.

British National Formulary, www.bnf.org.

Department of Health (2000) *Comprehensive Critical Care; A Review of Adult Critical Care Services*. The Stationery Office, London.

Morgan, R.J.M., Williams, F. and Wright, M.M. (1997) An early warning system for detecting developing critical illness. *Clinical Intensive Care*, **8**, 100.

Nursing and Midwifery Council (2002) *Code of Professional Conduct*. Nursing and Midwifery Council, London.

Royal College of Nursing (2005) *Agenda for Change: a guide to the new pay, terms and conditions in the NHS*. www.rcn.org.uk.

Subbe, C.P., Kruger, M., Rutherford, P. and Gemmel, L. (2001) Validation of modified early warning score in medical admissions. *Quality Journal of Medicine*, **94**, 521–526.

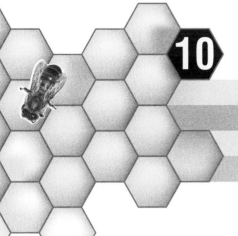

Exploring the nursing numeracy skills embedded in caring for a patient in a critical care context:

Mr Colin Morris

Learning outcomes

By the end of this chapter you should be able to:

- Recognise where numbers are in the nursing care of patients such as Colin Morris

- Calculate in a variety of nursing-related contexts

- Use numeracy skills to explore the nursing care of Mr Colin Morris

Introduction

In order to explore some of the numeracy skills embedded in caring for patients in a critical care setting, this chapter introduces you to Mr Colin Morris.

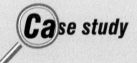

Case study

Colin Morris

Mr Colin Morris is a 56-year-old local government worker. He lives in a small village with his partner of six years, Libby (they are in the midst of planning their wedding, which is due to take place in three months' time). He has three children from his first marriage – Sam, 19, Abigail, 17 and Lisa, 13. They all live with their mother in a nearby town, and as well as seeing their father through the week they stay with him most weekends. Colin has been admitted to the Emergency Care Unit. He is complaining of substernal chest pain, which he describes as crushing in nature and radiates into his jaw. The pain began while he was at work; he has vomited undigested food twice and says he feels as though he is going to die. In the Emergency Care Unit Staff Nurse Jones is on duty and is allocated as Colin's primary nurse. She notices that Colin looks grey and ashen, with beads of perspiration on his skin. After welcoming Colin to the unit, making him comfortable and explaining why he has been admitted, she gains his consent to begin monitoring his cardiac function and his vital signs: BP 135/95mmHg, pulse 120bpm, respiratory rate 28, O_2 sats 97%, temperature 37°C. While doing this, she asks Colin some questions to explore the position and severity of his pain and to ascertain whether the analgesia given in the ambulance is having any effect. She also finds out that Libby, his partner, is Colin's next of kin and that Libby has been informed that Colin has been admitted to hospital. She also notices that Mr Morris is becoming a little breathless and has started to rub his left upper arm. When she

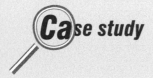

Case study

speaks to him to find out why he is rubbing his arm, he tells her he feels that his pain is getting worse again. The cardiac monitor shows that he is having short runs of ventricular tachycardia (VT) and occasional premature ventricular contractions (PVCs), BP 100/55mmHg, heart rate 120bpm, respiratory rate 25, O_2 sats 87%, temperature 37°C. He is given a bolus of Lidocaine (Lignocaine) 100 mg and an IV line is set up to give 500 ml of Lidocaine 0·2% in 5% glucose at a rate of 2 mg/min.

Over to you

Risk management

Using a volumetric pump, calculate the rate in ml/hr that you will have to key in to deliver the Lidocaine infusion.

Well done if you found the answer to be 60 ml/hr. If you have not got this answer, it could be that if you are using a calculator you have keyed in incorrect information at some point and you did not notice. When calculating information related to patient care it is extremely important that you get into the habit of checking the display on the calculator each time you enter data to ensure that the entry is correct. This should be done at every stage of the calculation. Try the calculation again, only this time check carefully that each number you key in is correct.

The solution that you have in this scenario is 500 ml of 0·2% Lidocaine in 5% glucose. Lidocaine, along with a small number of other medicines (e.g. Adrenaline/Epinephrine) is available in what are called percentage concentrations (see Chapter 4, p. 73–75). This is shorthand for saying how many grams there are in 100 ml of the solution. In a 1% solution there will be 1 g per 100 ml. So, in a 2% solution there will be 2 g in 100 ml (as you can see, the percentage changes but the volume never varies). Therefore, a 0·2% solution is shorthand for saying that there is 2 mg of Lidocaine in every 1 ml. The prescription is for 2 mg per minute. As a result, 1 ml has to be given every minute. You were asked for the rate in ml per hour so, as there are 60 minutes in an hour, you will have to multiply this by 60. The equation will look like this: $1 \times 60 = 60$ ml.

The equation for this calculation would be:

$$\text{dose} \times 60 = \text{ml/hr}$$

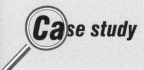

Case study

Mr Morris is also prescribed diamorphine 2 ml per hour of a 1 mg/ml solution with 0·9% sodium chloride.

Over to you

Risk management

The diamorphine available in the Emergency Department is in either 5 mg/1 ml or 10 mg/1 ml ampoules. Using a syringe driver that holds a 60 ml syringe, how will you make up the injection?

You want a solution that will deliver 1 mg per ml. Therefore, in a 60 ml syringe you will need 60 mg of diamorphine. You could use 6 × 10 mg ampoules of diamorphine. This would be 6 ml when drawn up into the syringe. In order to fill the syringe, you will have to draw up a further 54 ml of 0·9% sodium chloride (60 − 6 = 54). If you used 5 mg ampoules you would have to draw up 12 ampoules (60 mg/5 mg = 12); 12 ampoules would be 12 ml of fluid. Therefore, you would only need to draw up 48 ml of 0·9% sodium chloride (60 − 12 = 48).

Theory to practice

In this situation you need to understand:

- How to assess the patient's physiological condition as well as their pain so that evaluations of the patient's condition can be made
- The patho-physiological effects of myocardial infarction and the potential impacts on the cardiovascular system
- How a deteriorating physiological condition can be noticed by trends in vital signs, which are frequently accompanied by changes in the patient's skin and behaviour
- The psychological and sociological effects of myocardial infarction and the potential impact this may have on the patient and their family
- The way that fluid, electrolyte and acid/base balance can influence the heart and circulation.

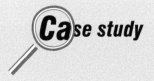
Case study

Case study continued

When she received the message to say that Colin was being taken to emergency admissions, Libby, Colin's partner, went straight to ECU from work. While sitting at Colin's bedside she noticed that there seemed to be insufficient staff available to meet patients' needs in the unit.

Theory to practice

You need to understand the roles and responsibilities that senior ward nurses have. It has been suggested that eventually nurses will be managing 70% of the overall NHS budget (Audit Commission 2001) and in order to achieve this the Department of Health has begun the process of delegating the control of ward and department budgets to ward managers. Consequently, as a qualified nurse, you will have some role to play in helping to balance the books. Managing a budget means controlling and auditing spending on staffing, supplies and equipment, as well as liaising with the Trust's financial team. It will also involve writing a business case for any new requirements.

As you are aware, all nursing staff are employed for a certain number of hours each week. Some nurses work full time (i.e. 37·5 hours per week) and others work part time (i.e. fewer than 37·5 hours per week). However, calculating ward-staffing levels by using the number of hours that are worked cumulatively per week by each nurse is unmanageable.

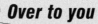

Over to you

Resource management

Why would using a cumulative calculation of hours worked by nurses on a ward not give you much information?

This information is limited as it would show the total numbers of hours worked but not the number of staff working those hours. Also, large numbers would be involved.

Calculations of ward staffing are usually done in wtes or whole-time equivalents. One whole-time equivalent equals 37·5 hours. This means that you could have one nurse or any number of nurses working those wte hours. Using this principle, you could have 36 nurses working an hour each and three nurses working a half-hour per week each. So ward staffing is set using a number of whole-time equivalent staff. In order to calculate the whole-time equivalents from actual staff hours, you will have to divide the actual hours worked by 37·5. It is usually the ward manager's responsibility to ensure that there are enough staff in post to fill the ward/unit staffing. The number of people the ward manager chooses to do this will vary from ward to ward as necessary.

Key points | Top tips

If you are using whole numbers, remember that in order to find a smaller amount you will have to use the skill of division.

Over to you

Resource management

The following is a list of Team A day staff and the hours that they work:

- Sr Smyth, band 6, 37·5 hrs
- Sr French, band 6, 24 hrs
- Ch/N Straker, band 6, 32 hrs
- S/N Jones, band 5, 37·5 hrs
- S/N West, band 5, 18 hrs
- S/N Wilmslow, band 5, 32 hrs

- S/N Darcy, band 5, 20 hrs
- S/N Moore, band 5, 25 hrs
- HCA Leeming, band 3, 37·5 hrs
- HCA Chester, band 2, 22·5 hrs
- HCA Murray, band 2, 36 hrs

Calculate the whole-time equivalents for each band of staff.

The whole-time equivalents per band are as follows:

- Band 6, 2·49 wte
- Band 5, 3·53 wte
- Band 3, 1 wte
- Band 2, 1·56 wte.

Skills checklist

The number skills required in this calculation are division and addition as well as those of rounding up and down. If you have been unable to do this calculation or if you have had difficulty doing it, ask yourself:

- Did I understand what I was being asked to do?
- Did I have the number skills to carry out this calculation?
- Were there any number principles/formulae I could have used?

Perform the calculation. Ask yourself:

- Is it correct?
- How did I feel about the process?
- What do I need to do now?

Your calculations should look like this.

Band 6: There is one full-time band 6, so that post is 37·5 hours (which = 1 wte), one of the part-time band 6 posts is 24 hours (which = $24 \div 37·5 = 0·64$ wte), one of the part-time band 6 posts is 32 hours (which = $32 \div 37·5 = 0·8533333$ wte, which rounded down is 0·85 wte).

To total the band 6 wtes, each of the wte hours must be added together. The calculation looks like this: $1 + 0·64 + 0·85$. Total = 2·49 wte.

You may have difficulty calculating figures that are presented horizontally, especially when stressed. People find it easier to calculate figures when they are presented in a **vertical** list. So in future when you are presented with **horizontal** lists of figures, turn the list into a vertical list. However, check carefully to make sure you do not make any transcription errors. If you are not sure how to do this, the band 5 calculations below are listed horizontally first and then vertically after that.

◦━ Keywords

Horizontal

On the same plane as the earth's horizon. A straight line on a flat or level surface, e.g.:

_____

at right angles to a vertical line

Vertical

A line perpendicular to the earth's horizon. At a 90° angle to a level flat surface, e.g.:

Band 5 – horizontal list: There is one full-time band 5 post, so that post is 37·5 hours (which = 1 wte); one of the part-time band 5 posts is 18 hours (which = $18 \div 37·5 = 0·48$); one of the part-time band 5 posts is 32 hours (which = $32/37·5 = 0·8533333$, which rounded down is 0·85); one of the part-time band 5 posts is 20 hours (which = $20 \div 37·5 = 0·53$); one of the part-time band 5 posts is 25 hours (which = $25 \div 37·5 = 0·66666$, which rounded up is 0·67). The total is $1 + 0·48 + 0·85 + 0·53 + 0·67 = 3·53$ wte.

Band 5 – vertical list: There is one full-time band 5 post so that post is 37·5 hours (which = 1 wte).

One of the part-time band 5 posts is 18 hours (which = $18 \div 37·5 = 0·48$).

One of the part-time band 5 posts is 32 hours (which = $32 \div 37·5 = 0·8533333$, which rounded down is 0·85).

One of the part-time band 5 posts is 20 hours (which = $20 \div 37·5 = 0·53$).

One of the part-time band 5 posts is 25 hours (which = $25 \div 37·5 = 0·66666$, which rounded up is 0·67).

Thus

1·0

0·48

0·85

0·53

0·67

Total = 3·53 wte.

Band 3: There is one full-time band 3 post so that post is 37·5 hours (which = 1 wte).

The total is 1 wte.

Band 2: One of the part-time band 2 posts is 22·5 hours (which = $22·5 \div 37·5 = 0·6$); one of the part-time band 2 posts is 36 hours (which = $36 \div 37·5 = 0·96$). Total = $0·6 + 0·96 = 1·56$ wte.

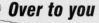

> ### Over to you
>
> #### Resource management
> Sister Jacobs is the unit manager and Staff Nurse Rogers is in the unit's Team B band 5. S/N Rogers has asked if she can reduce her hours from 32 to 24 per week. Team B's staffing for band 5s is 3·6 whole-time equivalents (wtes). The band 5 staffing establishment for Team B is currently: Staff Nurse Radcliffe working full time, Staff Nurse Rogers working 32 hours, Staff Nurse Blake working 28 hours, Staff Nurse Vary working 16 hours and Staff Nurse Vodusek working 21 hours.

> ### Over to you
>
> #### Resource management
> In order to comply with Staff Nurse Rogers' request, Sr Jacobs will need to make a calculation. What will this calculation be? What will the number of hours be, and what will the wte be?

Sr Jacobs will have to work out the difference in whole-time equivalents between the 32 hours that Staff Nurse Rogers works now and the 24 hours that she would like to work: 32 hours – 24 hours = 8 hours; $8 \div 37\cdot5 = 0\cdot21$ (rounded down).

> ### Over to you
>
> #### Resource management
> As the staffing establishment is calculated in whole-time equivalents, what are the whole-time equivalents of each of the Team B staff nurses?

The whole-time equivalents are:
S/N Radcliffe $37\cdot5 = 1\cdot0$ wte
S/N Rogers $32 \div 37\cdot5 = 0\cdot85$ wte
S/N Blake $28 \div 37\cdot5 = 0\cdot75$ wte
S/N Vary $16 \div 37\cdot5 = 0\cdot43$ wte
S/N Vodusek $21 \div 37\cdot5 = 0\cdot56$ wte

> ### Over to you
>
> #### Resource management
> What possibilities can you suggest so that Staff Nurse Rogers can reduce her hours?

The possibilities include:

- Any of the other part-time staff nurses could pick up all of the extra eight hours
- The eight hours could be split between any of the other part-time staff nurses
- Sr Jacobs could employ another staff nurse for eight hours a week (0·21 wte).

Skills checklist

The number skills required in this calculation are division and subtraction, as well as those of rounding up and rounding down. If you have been unable to do this calculation or if you have had difficulty in doing it, ask yourself:

- Did I understand what I was being asked to do?
- Did I have I the number skills to carry out this calculation?
- Were there any number principles/formulae I could have used?

Perform the calculation. Ask yourself:

- Is it correct?
- How did I feel about the process?
- What do I need to do now?

Theory to practice

Working in situations such as this you need to understand how to calculate whole-time equivalents, but you also need to understand what skills the staff should have in order to deliver an efficient and cost-effective service. If you do not fully understand skill mix, you may find the following articles helpful: Crossan, F. and Ferguson, D. (2005) Exploring nursing skill mix: a review. *Journal of Nursing Management,* **13**, 356–362; and Currie, V. *et al.* (2005) Relationship between quality of care, staffing levels, skill mix and nurse autonomy: a literature review. *Journal of Advanced Nursing,* **51**(1), 73–82.

Over to you

Resource management

The critical care unit has predicted annual costs of £619,000. What would the unit costs be if the monthly outgoings increased by 8%?

> ### *Theory to practice*
>
> Before working out a calculation like this, it is important that you understand how the monthly outgoings will be increased. It is important to clarify whether the monthly outgoings will increase month by month by 8% or whether they will increase over the year by 8%. The difference in the budget could be substantial and would result in a massive unexpected overspend. If you are unfamiliar with NHS financial accountancy you can clarify your understanding with the Trust's financial team. You may find this resource helpful: Brown, S. and Green, A. (eds) (2004) *Introductory guide to NHS finance in the UK.* Healthcare Financial Management Association, Bristol.

First, you would have to find out whether the costs would increase on a month-by-month basis or by 8% per month. If the outgoings increase month-on-month by 8%, the calculation for the first month will be £619,000 ÷ 12 × 8%. The calculation will appear as follows:

$$\frac{£619,000}{12} = 51,583 \times \frac{8}{100} = £4,126 \cdot 64$$

No doubt you will have remembered that this is per month, so every month the outgoing will increase by another 8%. So by the end of the financial year the extra 8% month on month will mean extra spending of £129,888. You can work this out by adding the 8% increase for the first month on to the monthly outgoings:

$$\text{First monthly outgoing} = \frac{£619,000}{12} = 51,583$$

Then add an extra 8% on to this amount. For every month after this you will have to add 8% on to the increased amount of outgoings. So, for example, the month-on-month increased outgoings will be as follows:

Month 1, the first increased monthly outgoings (£51,583) plus 8% which is £51,583 + £4,126 = £55,710

Month 2, the second month's increased outgoings = £55,710 + 8% = £60,167

Month 3, the third month's increased outgoings = £60,167 + 8% = £64,981

Month 4, the fourth month's increased outgoings = £64,981 + 8% = £70,180

Month 5, the fifth month's increased outgoings = £70,180 + 8% = £75,795

Month 6, the sixth month's increased outgoings = £75,795 + 8% = £81,859

Month 7, the seventh month's increased outgoings = £81,859 + 8% = £88,408

Month 8, the eighth month's increased outgoings = £88,408 + 8% = £95,481

Month 9, the ninth month's increased outgoings = £95,481 + 8% = £103,120

Month 10, the tenth month's increased outgoings = £103,120 + 8% = £111,370

Month 11, the eleventh month's increased outgoings = £111,370 + 8% = £120,280

Month 12, the twelfth month's increased outgoings = £120,280 + 8% = £129,903.

If you did not get these answers it could be because each of the totals above have been rounded up. Each time the figures are rounded up they become bigger, so when they are continually rounded up (in this example 12 times) the final figure will be considerably larger and therefore not particularly accurate. However, they will give a good approximation. The opposite applies when rounding down.

Key points **Top tips**

- Be careful when rounding figures
- Ensure that you understand what calculation you have to do.

As you can see, the costs are rising very quickly. If this continues, the final cost at the end of month 12 will be £1,057,254 In order to find out how much the year's total outgoings would be in this situation, each of the monthly totals will have to be added together. Calculating the costs this way means that the outgoings will be almost twice as much as the predicted costs of £619,000.

By comparison, if the outgoings were to increase by 8% per month across the whole year, the calculation would look like this:

One month's extra spend would be:

$$\frac{£619,000}{12} \times \frac{8}{100} = £4,126 \cdot 64$$

12 months' extra spend would be:

£4,127 × 12 = £49,524

Add this to the previous annual costs to find the new annual costs:

£619,000 + £49,524 = £668,524

To calculate the new monthly outgoings, divide the new annual costs by 12:

$$\frac{£668,524}{12} = £55,710$$

> ### Over to you
>
> **Resource management**
> Calculate the difference between the predicted total yearly amounts of spending at an increase of 8% per month, and a year with the 8% month-on-month increased spending.

If the outgoings were to increase by 8% per month across the whole year, the annual the outgoings would be £685,840. If the outgoings were to rise by 8% month-on-month, the outgoings would be £1,057,254. The difference between the two (£1,057,254 − £668,524) is £388,730.

In reality you would only expected to use one method or the other, but comparing both methods demonstrates clearly that you must understand what you are being asked to do.

> **Key points** **Top tips**
>
> It is important that you are sure about what you are being asked to do.

> ### Skills checklist
>
> The number skills required in this calculation are division, multiplication and addition, as well as those related to percentages. If you have been unable to do this calculation or if you have had difficulty doing it, ask yourself:
>
> ● Did I understand what I was being asked to do?
> ● Did I have the number skills to carry out this calculation?
> ● Were there any number principles/formulae I could have used?
>
> Perform the calculation. Ask yourself:
>
> ● Is it correct?
> ● How did I feel about the process?
> ● What do I need to do now?

Key points **Top tips**

- Dividing one number with another number will give an answer to a calculation that is smaller than the original numbers. Division is therefore another means of subtraction
- Conversely, multiplying numbers will give an answer that is larger than the original numbers. In other words, multiplication is another form of addition.

Over to you

Resource management

As has already been indicated, the critical care unit where Colin is being cared for has an annual budget of £619,000. A print-out of the budget on 30 August shows that the expenditure to date is £309,500. What percentage of your budget has been spent to date?

Good work if your calculation showed 50%. Some of you will have been able to see straight away that £309,500 is half of £619,000 and that half in percentage terms is 50%. If you did not get this answer, then take a few minutes to think about what you were asked to do. The expenditure is less than the total amount; a rough estimation therefore would be about half as much (£300,000 is half as much as £600,000). So this calculation involves dividing the expenditure to date (£309,500) by the annual budget (£619,000). As we need a percentage, and this will mean a larger figure, the figure will have to be multiplied by 100. This is how the calculation should look:

$$\frac{\text{Expenditure to date}}{\text{Annual budget}} \times 100$$

So, for this example the figures would be:

$$\frac{309,500}{619,000} \times 100$$

Do not forget about BODMAS – the division must be done before the multiplication. First, cancel out the two noughts from both the numerator and denominator, then one of the noughts in the 100 and the remaining nought in the denominator. Divide 309,500 by 619,000 which gives an answer of a half, which is 50%:

$$\frac{309,\cancel{500}}{619,\cancel{000}} \times 10\cancel{0} = \frac{309,50}{619} = \frac{1}{2} \quad 50\%$$

Over to you

Resource management

In the previous example you calculated that the unit had spent 50% of its annual budget to 30 August. Given the same rate of spending, will there be an overspend or underspend in the ward budget at the end of the financial year?

Nice work if you said there would be an overspend. If you did not get this answer, let us think about what you were asked to do. You were asked to predict whether there would be an over- or underspend by the end of the financial year. In your calculation did you remember that the financial year runs from 1 April until 31 March? You know what the spending is for 1 April to 30 August, which is five months. This means that there are seven months left in the financial year in question.

Theory to practice

Working in situations like this, you need to understand that if the unit continues to spend at the same rate, the money will run out at the end of February. Consequently, action needs to be taken now to identify where any overspend has taken place and identify savings that would bring the budget in on target. This will mean analysing the budget statement carefully to identify which areas are overspent and which are underspent. In order to bring the budget in on target you will need to examine any areas of cost that are both controllable and predictable.

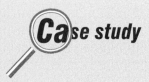

Case study

Case study continued

The critical care unit is asked to collect a lot of data in relation to the work that it carries out. Data that is routinely collected about the activities of the unit is related to the age group of the patients cared for in that unit. The ages of the patients who were admitted to the unit in the last month are:

6 patients aged 88 years,	3 patients aged 75 years,	4 patients aged 84 years,
3 patients aged 72 years,	5 patients aged 79 years,	6 patients aged 78 years,
3 patients aged 70 years,	4 patients aged 21 years,	2 patients aged 19 years,
2 patients aged 68 years,	1 patient aged 60 years,	3 patients aged 42 years,
2 patients aged 69 years,	4 patients aged 71 years,	7 patients aged 18 years,
6 patients aged 82 years,	3 patients aged 85 years,	6 patients aged 77 years,
2 patients aged 86 years,	5 patients aged 81 years,	5 patients aged 17 years,
6 patients aged 89 years,	3 patients aged 91 years,	3 patients aged 76 years.

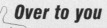

Over to you

Resource management
What is the average age of the patients?

Well done if you calculated the average age to be 67 years, or 66·765 years before you rounded up. If you did not get 67 as the answer, check your calculation again. If you are having difficulties, this may be for a number of reasons – see our Skills checklist and Top tip on pages 164–5. This type of average is what mathematicians/statisticians call the **mean**.

⊶ Keywords

Mean
One type of average. It is the total of the quantities divided by how many there are

Theory to practice

The number skills required in this calculation are addition and division. If you have been unable to do this calculation or if you have had difficulty in doing this calculation, ask yourself:

● Did I understand what I was being asked to do?

● Did I have the number skills to carry out this calculation?

● Were there any number principles/formulae I could have used?

Perform the calculation. Ask yourself:

● Is it correct?

● How did I feel about the process?

● What do I need to do now?

The mean is found by dividing the sum of the measurements by the total number of measurements. To work out the mean, you need to add the ages of the patients together. The mean will be a smaller amount than the sum of the total ages, which are 6,276. In order to get a smaller answer, you then have to divide 6,276 by the total number of patients (94). The equation will therefore look like this:

$6276 \div 94 = 66\cdot765$, or rounded up to 67 years

You will have noticed that even though the majority of these patients seem to be in their seventies and eighties, the mean age is in the sixties. How representative of the patient group is a mean age of 67?

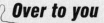

> ## Over to you
>
> ### Resource management
> Take a few moments to explain why you think that the mean age is 67 when most patients seem to be older than that.

Well done if you said that the mean age could be **skewed** because there are only a few numbers that are either large or small in comparison to the rest of the numbers.

> ## Over to you
>
> ### Resource management
> Is 67 years of age representative of the age group of the patients you would be caring for if you were looking after Colin?

No, it is not really, is it? The patients cared for in the unit in the past month seem to be predominantly in their seventies and eighties.

> ## Over to you
>
> ### Resource management
> What could the implications be of using the mean age in this situation?

Older people often have different care needs than younger people (Department of Health 2001). Older people are more likely than younger people to have multiple pathologies, which would mean that older people will also tend to have more complex care and treatment needs. The age of the patients could therefore have an impact on calculating staffing requirements. The unit should have staff in post who have the necessary knowledge skills and attitudes to care for older people. Therefore, using the mean in this situation would not give a true reflection of the extra staffing requirements and costs that are needed to care for the complex needs of older people.

Over to you

Resource management
Which type of average would be most appropriate to use to find a more representative sample of the age of these patients?

Keywords

Median
A way of expressing an average. When you arrange all the numbers in ascending order, the median is the middle number

It would be preferable to use the **median** to reflect a truer picture of the age group of these patients.

Over to you

Resource management
What would be the median age of the above group of patients?

The median age would be 77 years. You can find the median by listing the ages in ascending order, so the ages of this group of patients will look like this: 17, 17, 17, 17, 17, 18, 18, 18, 18, 18, 18, 18, 19, 19, 21, 21, 21, 21, 42, 42, 42, 60, 68, 68, 69, 69, 70, 70, 70, 71, 71, 71, 71, 72, 72, 72, 75, 75, 75, 76, 76, 76, 77, 77, 77, 77, 77, 77, 78, 78, 78, 78, 78, 78, 79, 79, 79, 79, 79, 81, 81, 81, 81, 81, 82, 82, 82, 82, 82, 82, 84, 84, 84, 84, 85, 85, 85, 86, 86, 88, 88, 88, 88, 88, 88, 89, 89, 89, 89, 89, 89, 91, 91, 91. There are 94 numbers in this list, so the median is halfway between the 47th and 48th numbers, i.e. number 77.

Over to you

Resource management
There is another form of average that could be used here. What is it? Would it be representative of the patients using the critical care unit in this situation?

Keywords

Mode
This is also an average. It is the most frequently occurring number in a set of numbers (data)

The form of average known as the **mode** could be used. However, it will not give a true representation of the ages of these patients, so it would be inappropriate to use in this situation.

If you look at the data set (list of numbers) for this group of patients, you will see that the most frequently occurring number or age is 18 years. This is because there were seven patients in this age group, which makes this age group the most frequently occurring. Here is the data set again:

6 patients aged 88 years,   3 patients aged 75 years,
4 patients aged 84 years,   3 patients aged 72 years,
5 patients aged 79 years,   6 patients aged 78 years,
3 patients aged 70 years,   4 patients aged 21 years,
2 patients aged 19 years,   2 patients aged 68 years,
1 patient aged 60 years,   3 patients aged 42 years,
2 patients aged 69 years,   4 patients aged 71 years,
7 patients aged 18 years,   6 patients aged 82 years,
3 patients aged 85 years,   6 patients aged 77 years,
2 patients aged 86 years,   5 patients aged 81 years,
5 patients aged 17 years,   6 patients aged 89 years,
3 patients aged 91 years,   3 patients aged 76 years.

You can see that using the mean would appear to be more representative of the patient group being cared for in the unit that month. This average figure would favour any argument to support strengthening skill mix and staffing not only to meet the more complex care needs of older people, but also to meet the targets of the NSF for Older People (2001).

The previous activities have focused on one of the key concepts of statistical thinking, namely the average. You will have encountered the word 'average' as it occurs frequently in everyday life. Common examples that you will have come across will be: average height, average weight, average wage and the average family. However, as the previous activities will have highlighted, the word 'average' is used to describe a representative value and there are a number of ways of finding such a representative.

The reason for this is that when we need to be able to describe the measurable aspect of an assortment of items (data) (e.g. height or weight) we are often confronted with some differences in the data (the items to be measured). The previous activities will have clearly demonstrated that what is usually referred to in everyday life as the average is, in fact, one of three different types of average: mean, median and mode.

Reflective activity

Consider how you feel about your understanding of the concepts of mean, median and mode. You might like to identify this as an area of continuing professional development in your Professional Portfolio. If you would like to do this, we suggest you read further about mean, median, mode and averages.

Rapid recap

Check your progress so far by working through each of the following points.

1. Provide an example of numeracy within this chapter which you might need to explain to a student nurse
2. Explain how this calculation would be relevant to a student nurse
3. Identify a source of help for those experiencing difficulties in some aspect of the calculation

If you have difficulty with more than one of these questions, read through the section again to refresh your understanding.

References

Audit Commission (2001) *Ward staffing (acute hospital portfolio, review of national findings, No. 3)*. London: Audit Commission.

Brown S. and Green A. (eds) (2004) *Introductory guide to NHS finance in the UK*. Healthcare Financial Management Association, Bristol.

Crossan, F. and Ferguson, D. (2005) Exploring nursing skill mix: a review. *Journal of Nursing Management*, **13**, 356–362.

Currie, V., Harvey, G., Wes, E., McKenna, H. and Keeney, S. (2005) Relationship between quality of care, staffing levels, skill mix and nurse autonomy: a literature review. *Journal of Advanced Nursing*, **51**(1), 73–82.

Department of Health (2001) *National Service Framework for Older People*. www.dh.qov.uk.

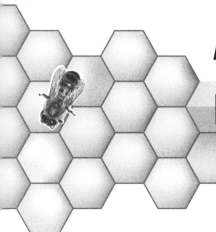

Appendix A

Rapid Recap – answers

Chapter 1

1. **Identify some areas in care delivery where we need to use objective measurements**

1. Some areas in care delivery where we need to use objective measurements are:
   - Clinical observations such as blood pressure, pulse, respiratory rate
   - Fluid balance
   - Measuring height and weight.

2. **Suggest two reasons why nurses might be concerned about their numeracy skills**

2. Reasons why nurses might be concerned about their numeracy skills are:
   - They do not undertake calculations on a regular basis
   - They have not been taught numeracy related to work
   - The general population is less numerate
   - They are unable to transfer their skills
   - They do not value their skills.

3. **Identify some current initiatives in nursing which will require a greater awareness of numeracy**

3. Some current initiatives in nursing which will require a greater awareness of numeracy are:
   - Prescribing
   - Greater use of technology
   - New roles
   - Expert patient initiative
   - Evidence-based practice.

4. **Identify the underpinning philosophy for this new approach to numeracy**

4. The underpinning philosophy for this new approach to numeracy is that: nurses should understand the calculations they are involved with; they should be able to recognise and use their numeracy experience in a range of contexts; learning numeracy ought to be related to the world of work; and it should build confidence and competence.

Chapter 2

1. **What term is used to describe the uncomfortable feelings that many people experience in relation to their numeracy skills?**

1. Maths anxiety is the term used to describe this.

2. **Stereotype threat is said to have an impact on many people's numerical abilities. What kind of effect does it have?**

2. Stereotype threat is said to inhibit people's perceptions of their abilities.

3. **List three factors that can affect the ability of adults to calculate**

3. Factors that can affect the ability of adults to calculate are:
   - Teachers' impatience
   - Heart-sink calculations
   - Stereotype threat
     Inability to transfer skills.

Chapter 3

1. What are the *four rules of arithmetic*?

1. The *four rules of arithmetic* are:
   - Addition
   - Subtraction
   - Multiplication
   - Division.

2. Identify some number systems which you can use in calculations

2. Examples of number systems that you can use in calculations are:
   - BODMAS
   - Formulae
   - Rounding up figures
   - Guestimate.

3. Identify Pólya's strategies for solving mathematical problems

3. Pólya's strategies for solving mathematical problems are:
   - Understand the problem
   - Use previous experience to plan
   - Carry out the plan
   - Check how believable the answer is.

4. Identify some learning strategies which relate to understanding and learning numbers

4. Some learning strategies which relate to understanding and learning about numbers are:
   - Experiential learning
   - Reflection
   - Problem solving.

Chapter 4

1. Explain the term vulgar fraction

1. The term vulgar fraction is defined as where the value of a number is expressed by placing one number *over* another number.

2. How would you convert a vulgar fraction to a decimal fraction?

2. You would convert a vulgar fraction to a decimal fraction by dividing the bottom number into the top number.

3. Give an example of a formula used to establish the drip rate for an intravenous infusion

3. Examples of formulae used to establish the drip rate for an intravenous infusion are:

$$\text{rate (drops per minute)} = \frac{\text{volume} \times \text{drop factor (60)}}{\text{time (in hours)} \times \text{minutes in an hour}}$$

$$\text{delivery rate (ml per hour)} = \frac{\text{volume (in ml)}}{\text{time (in hours)}}$$

4. Provide two examples of formulae which could be used for calculating the dose of an oral medication

4. Examples of formulae which could be used for calculating the dose of an oral medication are:

$$\text{dose} = \frac{\text{strength required} \times \text{stock volume}}{\text{strength available}}$$

$$\text{weight related doses} = \frac{\text{recommended dose (per kg)} \times \text{body weight (in kg)}}{\text{number of doses per day}}$$

Chapter 5

1. What do SI units denote?

1. SI units refer to units of measurement.

2. What is meant by the term 'derived' unit?

2. The term 'derived' unit refers to measurements that are more complex, and are made up of more than one base unit.

3. Why have SI units been adopted?

3. The reason for identifying and adopting SI units in Britain was primarily safety. As patients, staff and information travel between countries, it was important to make this as safe as possible.

4. **Give three prefixes which would be used to denote a small unit**

4. Prefixes which would be used to denote a small unit are:
   - deci
   - centi
   - milli
   - micro
   - nano.

Chapter 6

1. **Name the three elements of care inherent in the approach to nursing numeracy used here**

1. The three elements of care inherent in our approach to nursing numeracy are:
   - Care management
   - Resource management
   - Risk management.

2. **Identify the strategies used in the approach in this book**

2. The strategies used in this book are:
   - Skills checklist
   - Top tips
   - Theory to practice.

3. **Explain why the approach in this book fosters transferability of learning**

3. The authors' approach fosters transferability of learning because it involves problem-solving strategies.

4. **Discuss the benefits of this approach for your professional development**

4. The benefits of their approach are that it includes reflection. identification of strengths and weaknesses, and planning.

Chapter 7

1. **Provide an example of numeracy within this chapter that you may have to explain to the patient**

1. Examples of numeracy within this chapter, which you might need to explain to the patient, are:
   - Changes in medication

   - Imperial equivalence of metric data
   - Health promotion advice.

2. **Identify an example of calculation used in this patient's care**

2. Examples of calculation used in this patient's care are:
   - Estimating heart rate from ECG
   - CLASP score
   - Fluid loss
   - Body Mass Index
   - Prevalence
   - Medication dose change
   - Salt calculation.

3. **Explain how the calculation is relevant to this patient's care**

3. The relevance of this calculation to this patient's care is that it enables you to:
   - Collect and interpret assessment data
   - Resource allocation
   - Health promotion
   - Medication concordance.

4. **Identify a source of help for those experiencing difficulties in some aspect of calculation**

4. The following sources will help you if you are experiencing difficulties in some aspect of calculation:
   - www.bbc.co.uk/bitesize
   - www.learndirect.org.uk
   - www.bdadyslexia.org.uk
   - Henderson, A. (1998) Maths for the Dyslexic: A Practical *Guide*. David Fulton, London.

Chapter 8

1. **Provide an example of numeracy within this chapter which you might need to explain to the patient**

1. Insulin via pen in response to carbohydrates in the diet is an example of numeracy within this chapter which you might need to explain to the patient.

2. **Identify an example of calculation used in this patient's care**

2. Intravenous infusion is an example of calculation used in this patient's care.

3. **Explain how the calculation is relevant to this patient's care**

3. The calculation relates to the correction of ketoacidosis in this patient.

4. **Identify a source of help for those experiencing difficulties in some aspect of calculation**

4. Sources of help for those experiencing difficulties with this calculation are:
   - www.bdadyslexia.org.uk/dyscalculia.html
   - www.bbc.co.uk/skillswise/tutors/expertcolumn/dyscalculia/index.shtml.

Chapter 9

1. **Provide an example of numeracy within this chapter that you may have to explain to a student nurse**

1. Examples of numeracy within this chapter that you might have to explain to a student nurse are:
   - MEWS scoring
   - Raytec gauze counts
   - Estimating fluid loss
   - Drip rates
   - Measuring and recording fluid balance
   - Staffing and budgeting.

2. **Explain how this calculation would be relevant to a student nurse**

2. This calculation would be relevant to a student nurse in order to:
   - Assess and interpret physiological data
   - Maintain patient safety
   - Provide adequate resources.

3. **Identify a source of help for those experiencing difficulties in some aspect of the calculation**

3. Sources of help for those experiencing difficulties in some aspect of the calculation are as follows:
   - www.bbc.co.uk/bitesize
   - www.learndirect.org.uk
   - www.bdadyslexia.org.uk
   - Henderson, A. (1998) *Maths for the Dyslexic: A Practical Guide*. David Fulton, London.

Chapter 10

1. **Provide an example of numeracy within this chapter which you might need to explain to a student nurse**

1. Examples of numeracy within this chapter that you might have to explain to a student nurse are:
   - Medicine dosage calculation; drip rate
   - Staffing
   - Budgeting
   - Analysing statistical data.

2. **Explain how this calculation would be relevant to a student nurse**

2. This calculation would be relevant to a student nurse in order to ensure:
   - Patient safety
   - Care delivery
   - Resource management
   - Developing service provision.

3. **Identify a source of help for those experiencing difficulties in some aspect of the calculation**

3. Sources of help for those experiencing difficulties in some aspect of the calculation are as follows:
   - www.bbc.co.uk/bitesize
   - www.learndirect.org.uk
   - www.bdadyslexia.org.uk
   - Henderson, A. (1998) *Maths for the Dyslexic: A Practical Guide*. David Fulton, London.

Appendix B

Refreshers

Chapter 3

Over to you
Refresher – identifying the problem

a. How many different ways can you multiply two whole positive numbers together to make 32? Identify these

b. How many different pairs of whole positive numbers add up to 12? Identify these

Over to you
Refresher – arithmetic

Addition
a. $56 + 8 =$
b. $561 + 18 =$
c. $56{\cdot}1 + 10 =$
d. $56{\cdot}1 + 1{\cdot}8 =$
e. $56{\cdot}1 + 1{\cdot}8 + 19 + 0{\cdot}1 =$

Subtraction
a. $56 - 8 =$
b. $561 - 18 =$
c. $56{\cdot}1 - 10 =$
d. $56{\cdot}1 - 1{\cdot}8 =$
e. $56{\cdot}1 - 9{\cdot}5 - 48 =$

Multiplication
a. $56 \times 8 =$
b. $561 \times 18 =$
c. $56{\cdot}1 \times 10 =$
d. $56{\cdot}1 \times 1{\cdot}8 =$
e. $56 \times 8 \times 10 =$

Division
a. $56 \div 8 =$
b. $561 \div 18 =$
c. $56{\cdot}1 \div 10 =$
d. $56{\cdot}1 \div 1{\cdot}8 =$
e. $56 \div 8 \div 1{\cdot}4 =$

And all together . . .
a. $561 + 8 - 1{\cdot}8 \times 10 \div 1{\cdot}4 =$
b. $561 + 8 - (18 \times 10) =$

Chapter 4

Over to you
Refresher – using BODMAS

a. $31 - 7 \times 4 =$
b. $28 \times 8 - 17 =$
c. $14 \div 2 \times 7 =$
d. $24 + 49 \div 7 - 18 =$

Over to you
Refresher – adding and simplifying fractions

Check your understanding by adding, subtracting and, where appropriate, simplifying the following fractions

a. $\dfrac{7}{8} + \dfrac{5}{8} + \dfrac{1}{8} =$

b. $\dfrac{3}{11} + \dfrac{6}{11} + \dfrac{1}{11} =$

c. $\dfrac{5}{9} + \dfrac{1}{3} + \dfrac{4}{9} =$

d. $\dfrac{4}{21} + \dfrac{8}{21} + \dfrac{3}{7} =$

e. $\dfrac{5}{6} - \dfrac{3}{6} =$

f. $\dfrac{5}{18} - \dfrac{2}{9} =$

g. $\dfrac{5}{6} - \dfrac{4}{9} =$

h. $\dfrac{7}{16} + \dfrac{4}{16} - \dfrac{5}{8} =$

Over to you
Refresher – multiplying and simplifying fractions

Check your understanding by adding, subtracting and where appropriate simplifying fractions

a. $\dfrac{4}{7} \times \dfrac{5}{8} =$

b. $\dfrac{3}{12} \times \dfrac{8}{14} =$

c. $\dfrac{5}{9} \times \dfrac{8}{9} =$

d. $\dfrac{7}{11} \times \dfrac{4}{5} =$

Over to you
Refresher – dividing and simplifying fractions

a. $\dfrac{1}{3} \div \dfrac{1}{5} =$

b. $\dfrac{3}{7} \div \dfrac{3}{5} =$

c. $\dfrac{9}{17} \div \dfrac{10}{17} =$

d. $\dfrac{17}{21} \div \dfrac{9}{11} =$

Over to you
Refresher – changing vulgar fractions to decimal fractions

Change the following to decimal fractions

a. $\dfrac{2}{7} =$

b. $\dfrac{5}{4} =$

c. $\dfrac{8}{11} =$

d. $\dfrac{7}{8} =$

Over to you
Refresher – decimals
a. Write 444·44 in words
b. Express two thousand, two hundred and twenty in figures
c. Multiply 4·4 by 1,000
d. Divide 222·2 by 10.

Change the following to vulgar fractions, and simplify where possible:
a. 0·55 =
b. 0·72 =
c. 0·68 =
d. 0·09 =

Over to you
Refresher – ratios

Calculate the following ratios:
a. Four patients in the ward of 30 are ready for discharge – what is the ratio of patients ready for discharge to patients remaining?
b. Eight out of 24 beds are occupied – what is the ratio of occupied to empty beds?
c. There are six empty beds in a ward of 24 beds – what is the ratio of empty to occupied beds?
d. Of the 24 patients in the ward, three have the blood group AB – what is the ratio of patients with blood group AB to patients with another blood group?

Over to you

Refresher – percentages

Calculate the following percentages:
a. Six empty beds in a ward of 24 beds
b. Eighteen occupied beds in a ward of 24 beds
c. What percentage is 120 g of 200 g?
d. What percentage is 12 g of 150 g?

Over to you

Refresher – calculating oral medicines

You have a medicine dispensed as 400 milligrams in 20 millilitres. How many millilitres will you give if the doctor orders:
a. 80 milligrams?
b. 120 milligrams?
c. 50 milligrams?
d. 60 milligrams?

Over to you

Refresher – weight-related doses

A patient is to receive a dose of 5 mg per kg of body weight, per day, divided into four equal doses. What would be the individual dose for the following?
a. The patient weighs 64 kg
b. The patient weighs 72 kg
c. The patient weighs 76 kg
d. The patient weighs 80 kg.

Over to you

Refresher – drip rates

Calculate the drip rates for the following:
a. A patient is prescribed 1,000 ml of fluid over eight hours (20 drops per ml)
b. A patient is prescribed 500 ml of fluid over three hours (20 drops per ml)
c. A patient is prescribed 500 ml of fluid over eight hours (60 drops per ml)
d. A patient is prescribed 500 ml of fluid over six hours (60 drops per ml)

Chapter 5

Over to you

Refresher – units of measure

Write the following abbreviations or symbols in full:
a. 1 g =
b. 500 mg =
c. 450 mcg =
d. 2 ml =

How many milligrams in:
a. 1 gram =
b. 0·5 gram =
c. 0·02 gram =
d. 0·005 gram =

Express the following as grams and decimal parts of a gram:
a. 1,500 milligrams =
b. 750 milligrams =
c. 20 milligrams =
d. 1 milligram =

How many micrograms in:
a. 1 milligram =
b. 0·25 milligrams =
c. 0·05 milligrams =
d. 0·001 milligrams =

You have tablets strength 150 milligrams each. How many tablets will you give if the doctor orders:
a. 0·3 gram =
b. 0·45 gram =
c. 0·6 gram =
d. 0·15 gram =

You have tablets strength 10 milligrams each. How many tablets will you give if the doctor orders:
a. 0·05 gram =
b. 0·02 gram =
c. 0·1 gram =
d. 0·01 gram =

Over to you

Refresher – time

a. If an intravenous infusion of one litre sodium chloride commenced at 08.45 hours (8 hours 45 minutes) and finished at 13.50, how long has it taken to deliver the infusion?

State your answer in figures and words

b. Convert these times so that they refer to the 24-hour clock:

10.30 a.m.
10.30 p.m.

c. Convert these times from the 24-hour clock to a.m. or p.m.:

06.45
18.20

Over to you

Refresher – SI units

A patient is to receive an injection of cimetidine 120 mg by the intramuscular route. Ampoules on hand contain 200 mg/2 ml

a. To what do the terms mg and ml refer?

b. Calculate the dose required

A patient is prescribed 0·06 grams of codeine phosphate. Tablets on the ward contain 30 mg.

a. How many milligrams are there in a gram?

b. Which unit of measurement has the gram as its SI unit?

c. Convert the 0·06 grams into mg

d. Calculate the dose required

A boy is to receive an intravenous infusion of 400 ml glucose over eight hours. The barrel emits 60 drops per ml

a. To what does the abbreviation ml refer?

b. Calculate the correct drip rate in drops per minute

A child is prescribed Erythromycin. He is to receive 50 mg per kg of body weight per day, which is to split into four doses. The child weighs 12 kg

a. To what does the abbreviation kg refer?

b. Work out the daily dose for this child

c. Work out the individual dose for this child

A child is prescribed Digoxin elixir 0·08 mg. The stock solution contains 0·05 mg per ml.

a. How many micrograms are contained in a milligram?

b. Convert the 0·08 mg and the 0·05 mg to micrograms

c. Which unit of measurement has the millilitre as its SI unit?

d. Work out an individual dose of Digoxin for this child

A patient is prescribed 150 micrograms of levothyroxine. On hand are 0·05 mg tablets

a. To what does the abbreviation mg refer?

b. Work out the dose to be given

A patient is to receive an intravenous infusion of 1 litre of sodium chloride 0.9% over eight hours

a. How many millilitres in a litre?

b. Calculate the drip rate required in drops per minute (the drop factor is 20)

A patient is prescribed 9 mg of morphine intramuscularly. The ampoule contains 15 mg in 1 ml.

a. Work out the correct dose

Phenobarbitone 60 mg has been ordered. Stock ampoules contain 200 mg/ml

a. What volume should be given?

Appendix C
Refresher answers

Chapter 3

Over to you
Refresher – identifying the problem
a. **How many different ways can you multiply two whole positive numbers together to make 32? Identify these**

$1 \times 32, 2 \times 16, 4 \times 8,$

b. **How many different pairs of whole positive numbers add up to 12? Identify these**

$11 + 1, 10 + 2, 9 + 3, 8 + 4, 7 + 5, 6 + 6$

Over to you
Refresher – arithmetic

Addition
a. $56 + 8 = 64$
b. $561 + 18 = 579$
c. $56 \cdot 1 + 10 = 66 \cdot 1$
d. $56 \cdot 1 + 1 \cdot 8 = 57 \cdot 9$
e. $56 \cdot 1 + 1 \cdot 8 + 19 + 0 \cdot 1 = 77$

Subtraction
a. $56 - 8 = 48$
b. $561 - 18 = 543$
c. $56 \cdot 1 - 10 = 46 \cdot 1$
d. $56 \cdot 1 - 1 \cdot 8 = 54 \cdot 3$
e. $56 \cdot 1 - 9 \cdot 5 - 48 = -1 \cdot 4$

Multiplication
a. $56 \times 8 = 448$
b. $561 \times 18 = 10,098$
c. $56 \cdot 1 \times 10 = 561$
d. $56 \cdot 1 \times 1 \cdot 8 = 100 \cdot 98$
e. $56 \times 8 \times 10 = 4,480$

Division
a. $56 \div 8 = 7$
b. $561 \div 18 = 31 \cdot 1666\ldots$
c. $56 \cdot 1 \div 10 = 5 \cdot 61$
d. $56 \cdot 1 \div 1 \cdot 8 = 31 \cdot 1666\ldots$
e. $56 \div 8 \div 1 \cdot 4 = 5$

And all together . . .
a. $561 + 8 - 1 \cdot 8 \times 10 \div 1 \cdot 4 = 556 \cdot 143$
b. $561 + 8 - (18 \times 10) = 389$

Chapter 4

Over to you
Refresher – using BODMAS
a. $31 - 7 \times 4 = 31 - (7 \times 4) = 3$
b. $28 \times 8 - 17 = (28 \times 8) - 17 = 207$
c. $14 \div 2 \times 7 = (14 \div 2) \times 7 = 49$
d. $24 + 49 \div 7 - 18 = 24 + (49 \div 7) - 18 = 13$

Over to you
Refresher – adding and simplifying fractions

Check your understanding by adding, subtracting and, where appropriate, simplifying the following fractions

a. $\dfrac{7}{8} + \dfrac{5}{8} + \dfrac{1}{8} = \dfrac{13}{8}$ or $1\dfrac{5}{8}$

b. $\dfrac{3}{11} + \dfrac{6}{11} + \dfrac{1}{11} = \dfrac{10}{11}$

c. $\dfrac{5}{9} + \dfrac{1}{3} + \dfrac{4}{9} = \dfrac{12}{9} = 1\dfrac{3}{9} = 1\dfrac{1}{3}$

d. $\dfrac{4}{21} + \dfrac{8}{21} + \dfrac{3}{7} = \dfrac{21}{21} = 1$

e. $\dfrac{5}{6} - \dfrac{3}{6} = \dfrac{2}{6} = \dfrac{1}{3}$

f. $\dfrac{5}{18} - \dfrac{2}{9} = \dfrac{1}{18}$

g. $\dfrac{5}{6} - \dfrac{4}{9} = \dfrac{7}{18}$

h. $\dfrac{7}{16} + \dfrac{4}{16} - \dfrac{5}{8} = \dfrac{1}{16}$

Over to you
Refresher – multiplying and simplifying fractions

Check your understanding by adding, subtracting and where appropriate simplifying fractions

a. $\dfrac{4}{7} \times \dfrac{5}{8} = \dfrac{20}{56} = \dfrac{5}{14}$

b. $\dfrac{3}{12} \times \dfrac{8}{14} = \dfrac{24}{168} = \dfrac{1}{7}$

c. $\dfrac{5}{9} \times \dfrac{8}{9} = \dfrac{40}{81}$

d. $\dfrac{7}{11} \times \dfrac{4}{5} = \dfrac{28}{55}$

Over to you
Refresher – dividing and simplifying fractions

a. $\dfrac{1}{3} \div \dfrac{1}{5} = 1\dfrac{2}{3}$

b. $\dfrac{3}{7} \div \dfrac{3}{5} = \dfrac{5}{7}$

c. $\dfrac{9}{17} \div \dfrac{10}{11} = \dfrac{99}{170}$

d. $\dfrac{17}{21} \div \dfrac{9}{11} = \dfrac{187}{189}$

Over to you
Refresher – changing vulgar fractions to decimal fractions

Change the following to decimal fractions

a. $\dfrac{2}{7} = 0.286$

b. $\dfrac{5}{4} = 1.25$

c. $\dfrac{8}{11} = 0.7272$ recurring

d. $\dfrac{7}{8} = 0.875$

Over to you
Refresher – decimals
a. **Write 444·44 in words**
   Four hundred and forty-four point four four
b. **Express two thousand, two hundred and twenty in figures**
   2,220
c. **Multiply 4·4 by 1,000**
   4,400
d. **Divide 222·2 by 10**
   22·22

Change the following to vulgar fractions, and simplify where possible:
a. 0·55 = 55/100 = 11/20
b. 0·72 = 72/100 = 18/25
c. 0·68 = 68/100 = 34/50 = 17/25
d. 0·09 = 9/100

Over to you
Refresher – ratios

Calculate the following ratios:
a. **Four patients in the ward of 30 are ready for discharge – what is the ratio of patients ready for discharge to patients remaining?**
   4:26 = 2:13
b. **Eight out of 24 beds are occupied – what is the ratio of occupied to empty beds?**
   8:16 = 1:2

c. There are six empty beds in a ward of 24 beds – what is the ratio of empty to occupied beds?

6:18 = 1:3

d. Of the 24 patients in the ward, three have the blood group AB – what is the ratio of patients with blood group AB to patients with another blood group?

3:21 = 1:7

Over to you

Refresher – percentages

Calculate the following percentages:

a. Six empty beds in a ward of 24 beds

$$6 \times \frac{100}{24} = 25\%$$

b. Eighteen occupied beds in a ward of 24 beds

$$18 \times \frac{100}{24} = 75\%$$

c. What percentage is 120 g of 200 g?

$$120 \times \frac{100}{200} = 60\%$$

d. What percentage is 12 g of 150 g?

$$12 \times \frac{100}{150} = 8\%$$

Over to you

Refresher – calculating oral medicines

You have a medicine dispensed as 400 milligrams in 20 millilitres. How many millilitres will you give if the doctor orders:

a. **80 milligrams?**

4 millilitres

b. **120 milligrams?**

6 millilitres

c. **50 milligrams?**

2·5 millilitres

d. **60 milligrams?**

3 millilitres

Over to you

Refresher – weight-related doses

A patient is to receive a dose of 5 mg per kg of body weight, per day, divided into four equal doses. What would be the individual dose for the following?

a. **The patient weighs 64 kg**

80 mg

b. **The patient weighs 72 kg**

90 mg

c. **The patient weighs 76 kg**

95 mg

d. **The patient weighs 80 kg**

100 mg

Over to you

Refresher – drip rates

Calculate the drip rates for the following:

a. **A patient is prescribed 1,000 ml of fluid over eight hours (20 drops per ml)**

42 dpm

b. **A patient is prescribed 500 ml of fluid over three hours (20 drops per ml)**

56 dpm

c. **A patient is prescribed 500 ml of fluid over eight hours (60 drops per ml)**

63 dpm

d. **A patient is prescribed 500 ml of fluid over six hours (60 drops per ml)**

84 dpm

Chapter 5

Over to you

Refresher – units of measure

Write the following abbreviations or symbols in full:

a. 1 g = 1 gram

b. 500 mg = 500 milligrams

c. 450 mcg = 450 micrograms

d. 2 ml = 2 millilitres

How many milligrams in:

a. 1 gram = 1,000

b. 0·5 gram = 500

c. 0·02 gram = 20

d. 0·005 gram = 5

Express the following as grams and decimal parts of a gram:
a. 1500 milligrams = 1·5
b. 750 milligrams = 0·75
c. 20 milligrams = 0·02
d. 1 milligram = 0·001

How many micrograms in:
a. 1 milligram = 1,000
b. 0·25 milligrams = 250
c. 0·05 milligrams = 50
d. 0·001 milligrams = 1

You have tablets strength 150 milligrams each, how many tablets will you give if the doctor orders:
a. 0·3 gram = 2 tablets
b. 0·45 gram = 3 tablets
c. 0·6 gram = 4 tablets
d. 0·15 gram = 1 tablets

You have tablets strength 10 milligrams each, how many tablets will you give if the doctor orders:
a. 0·05 gram = 5 tablets
b. 0·02 gram = 2 tablets
c. 0·1 gram = 10 tablets
d. 0·01 gram = 1 tablet

Over to you
Refresher – time
a. **If an intravenous infusion of one litre sodium chloride commenced at 08.45 hours (8 hours 45 minutes) and finished at 13.50, how long has it taken to deliver the infusion?**
   State your answer in figures and words
   13.50 – 08.45 = 5.05
   Five hours and five minutes
b. **Convert these times so that they refer to the 24-hour clock:**
   10.30 a.m.
   10.30 hours
   10.30 p.m.
   22.30 hours
c. **Convert these times from the 24-hour clock to a.m. or p.m.:**
   06.45
   6.45 a.m.
   18.20
   6.20 p.m.

Over to you
Refresher – SI units

A patient is to receive an injection of cimetidine 120 mg by the intramuscular route. Ampoules on hand contain 200 mg/2 ml
a. **To what do the terms mg and ml refer?**
   Milligram and millilitre
b. **Calculate the dose required**
   1·2 ml

A patient is prescribed 0·06 grams of codeine phosphate. Tablets on the ward contain 30 mg
a. **How many milligrams are there in a gram?**
   1,000
b. **Which unit of measurement has the gram as its SI unit?**
   Mass
c. **Convert the 0·06 grams into mg**
   60 milligrams
d. **Calculate the dose required**
   2 tablets

A boy is to receive an intravenous infusion of 400 ml glucose over eight hours. The barrel emits 60 drops per ml
a. **To what does the abbreviation ml refer?**
   Millilitre
b. **Calculate the correct drip rate in drops per minute**
   50 dpm

A child is prescribed Erythromycin. He is to receive 50 mg per kg of body weight per day, which is to split into four doses. The child weighs 12 kg
a. **To what does the abbreviation kg refer?**
   Kilogram
b. **Work out the daily dose for this child**
   600 mg
c. **Work out the individual dose for this child**
   150 mg

A child is prescribed Digoxin elixir 0·08 mg. The stock solution contains 0·05 mg per ml
a. **How many micrograms are contained in a milligram?**
   1,000

b. **Convert the 0·08 mg and the 0·05 mg to micrograms**

80 micrograms and 50 micrograms respectively

c. **Which unit of measurement has the millilitre as its SI unit?**

Volume

d. **Work out an individual dose of Digoxin for this child**

1·6 ml

A patient is prescribed 150 micrograms of levothyroxine. On hand are 0·05 mg tablets.

a. **To what does the abbreviation mg refer?**

Milligram

b. **Work out the dose to be given**

3 tablets

A patient is to receive an intravenous infusion of 1 litre of sodium chloride 0.9% over eight hours

a. **How many millilitres in a litre?**

1,000 ml

b. **Calculate the drip rate required in drops per minute (the drop factor is 20)**

42

A patient is prescribed 9 mg of morphine intramuscularly. The ampoule contains 15 mg in 1 ml

a. **Work out the correct dose**

0·6 ml

Phenobarbitone 60 mg has been ordered. Stock ampoules contain 200 mg/ml

a. **What volume should be given?**

0·3 ml

Appendix D
Other answers

Chapter 4

Su Doku

1. The 'easy' answers

9	4	8	6	7	2	1	3	5
5	3	7	9	1	4	6	8	2
6	1	2	3	5	8	9	7	4
7	5	1	2	4	6	8	9	3
2	8	4	1	9	3	5	6	7
3	9	6	7	8	5	4	2	1
1	6	9	5	3	7	2	4	8
8	7	5	4	2	9	3	1	6
4	2	3	8	6	1	7	5	9

2. The 'medium' answers

3	1	4	9	8	2	7	5	6
5	8	7	4	1	6	3	2	9
9	6	2	7	5	3	1	4	8
8	9	5	3	2	4	6	7	1
2	7	1	8	6	9	5	3	4
6	4	3	5	7	1	8	9	2
1	5	9	6	4	7	2	8	3
7	3	6	2	9	8	4	1	5
4	2	8	1	3	5	9	6	7

3. The 'difficult' answers

9	7	3	6	2	5	1	4	8
5	4	6	8	1	7	9	2	3
1	8	2	3	4	9	5	7	6
8	3	1	9	6	2	7	5	4
6	9	5	1	7	4	8	3	2
7	2	4	5	8	3	6	1	9
4	1	9	7	3	6	2	8	5
2	6	7	4	5	8	3	9	1
3	5	8	2	9	1	4	6	7

Over to you

Identify two terms that might be used for each of the following:

1. Subtraction

1. Subtraction: minus, take away, difference

2. Multiplication

2. Multiplication: times, product

3. Division

3. Division: share, fraction, quotient.

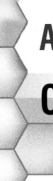

Appendix E

Count board blood loss answers

Packs (15 g)			Mops (10 g)		
Number of packs	Running total	Blood loss (ml) Running total	Number of mops	Running total	Blood loss (ml) Running total
6	6	904	4	40	60
5	11	165	2	6	90
3	14	210	3	9	100
7	21	315	1	10	
2	23	345			
4	27	405			
5	32	480			
3	35	525			
7	42	630			
9	51	765			
4	55	825			
6	61	915			
7	68	1,020			
3	71	1,065			

If your answers are different from this, check whether you remembered that each 15 g (dry weight) pack would weigh approximately 30 g when fully saturated with blood, so each 15 g (dry weight) pack used and discarded weighs 30 g, as it will have absorbed 15 ml of blood. The same principle applies for the log mop.

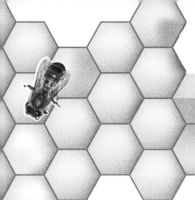

Appendix F

Fluid balance chart answers

FLUID BALANCE CHART

Name ......Gina Lloyd...................... Hospital Number 123zz45......... **Date** ...1.9.06............

Time	IV Line 1 Flagyl	IV Line 2 Cefuroxime	IV Line 3	Oral	Running Total	Drain 1	Drain 2	Urine	Running Total
0800	110	100	Packed Cells 125		335	150	125	32	307
0900			125		460	130	120	36	593
1000			125		585	132	120	36	881
1100			125		710	130	120	40	1171
1200			0.9%Sodium Chloride 125		835	130	115	41	1457
1300			125		900	130	115	45	1747
1400			125		1085	126	115	45	2033
1500			125		1210	46	6 8	45	2192
1600	100	100	125		1545	24	4 8	45	2309
1700			5% Glucose 125	30	1700	20	2 4	45	2398
1800			125	30	1855			50	2448
1900			125	30	2010	10	5	50	2513
2000			125	30	2165			45	2558
2100			125	60	2505			40	2598
2200			125	60	2630			40	2638
2300			125		2965			38	2676
2400	110	100	125		3150			42	2718
0100			125	60	3275			44	2762
0200			100		3400			40	2802
0300			Hartmann's Solution 125		3400			58	2860
0400			125		3525			65	2925
0500			125		3650			62	2987
0600			125		3775			68	3055
0700			125		3930			60	3155
Totals	330	300	3000	300	3930	1028	975	1112	3155
								Insensible loss 500	
	TOTAL INTAKE: 3930						**TOTAL OUTPUT: 3615**		
					BALANCE: + 315				

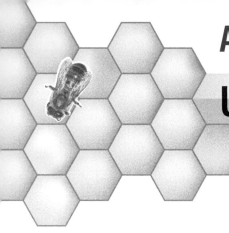

Appendix G

Using calculators

If you are using a calculator, you should be aware that there are three main types of calculator – not because it is interesting to know or that you could be asked a question in the pub quiz, but it is vital to know which type of calculator you are using so that you can understand some of the unexpected results that it may throw up. The main types of calculator are:

- **Four-function calculator**: This is a basic calculator and is adequate for most calculations. As well as the four functions (+, –, ×, ÷), it may have some other keys, most commonly the % key. Others may also have bracket and memory keys.
- **Scientific calculator**: This has more keys than a four-function calculator. This type usually has some trigonometric functions and memory keys, and they often have statistical functions.
- **Graphics calculator**: These calculators usually have a larger screen that displays each key press. They are scientific calculators but they also have graph-drawing functions and special statistical features.

As usual, it is not quite that straightforward, as within each of these three main types of calculator there can be a large variation between different brands and models. Consequently, you should spend some time getting to know how your calculator works and also how the ward calculator works.

The following activities have been included so that you can see some of the different ways that calculators can work and also understand why you need to be aware of the type of calculator you are using. These activities will raise your awareness of how differently calculators that use arithmetic logic work compared to those that use algebraic logic. If you have access to both a basic four-function calculator and a scientific calculator, try the activities with both calculators and note the results. You may be surprised by the differences.

For each of the following activities calculate in your head what the answers are and compare this with the final display on your calculator to see whether you are surprised with the results.

> ## Over to you
>
> Key this sequence into your calculator: 2 + 3 + = = (yes, this is the right sequence, it is not a typo; it will demonstrate something useful to you).

Yes, you are right, keying in 2 + 3 = will give the answer 5 on any calculator. On some calculators pressing an extra = will have no effect, but on some machines the calculator will add 3 again, and will keep adding three if you keep keying in =. Other calculators will add the two again and again. Some calculators do this if you key in the + twice rather than the =. For the technically minded of you, this is as a result of what is called the calculator's constant function. Now you can probably see why we included this exercise. It reinforces the need to be vigilant about your keystrokes when using a calculator in relation to your work. Cultivate a habit of checking the screen following each data entry to ensure you have entered what you think you have entered.

> ## Over to you
>
> Key in this sequence 2 + 3 × 4 =

Some calculators will show the answer as 14, while others will show the answer 20. Apparently, this depends on the order in which the calculator carries out the operations, and this depends on the type of logic it uses. Most scientific calculators use algebraic logic and consequently follow the rules of algebra and will carry out the multiplication before the addition (remember BODMAS, see Chapter 4, p. 61). However, calculators with arithmetical logic carry out the operations in the order that the keys are pressed. Consequently, 2 + 3 will be done first then × 5, thus giving the answer 20. Most four-function (basic) calculators have this kind of logic. This emphasises the importance of knowing which kind of calculator you are using, especially when calculating at work.

Calculating money

Some of the calculations you will be expected to do as a ward manager will involve budgeting. This often entails calculating money. There are some things that you need to be aware of when using a calculator to calculate money. This is also useful to know when you are trying to keep tabs on your own personal budget.

Over to you

Each item of wound dressing supplies has been costed as follows:
£12·50, £2·25, 75p, £28, 6p, £1·38
Using your calculator find out the total cost of these items.

Although this seems to be a straightforward calculation, you need to be careful that you are working either in pounds or pence. If you are working in pounds, then 75p should be entered as 0·75 and 6p as 0·06. Adding these to the amounts that are already expressed in pounds will give you an answer of £44·94.

Working out percentages using a calculator

While many calculators do have a percentage key, there is no need to use one if you remember that the word percentage means 'out of a hundred' and that you can think of the word 'of' in percentage as a multiplication.

Over to you

You read that 12% of patients taking a particular medicine develop DVT. The sample population was 4,789. How many patients in the sample population actually developed a DVT?

Well done if you answered 574. If you did not get his answer, check carefully that you have entered the calculation correctly, i.e. 12 ÷ 100 × 4,789. You will have noticed that the calculator gives the answer as 574·68. We have never met 0·68 of a person, so when we are using statistics that draw on numbers to represent people, we have to use whole numbers.

Conclusion

As a result of the previous activities you will have learnt some simple rules so that you can avoid making errors when entering calculations into a calculator. These rules are:

- Before starting any new calculation get into the habit of pressing the 'clear' key
- After entering every number check the display to confirm that the number you have entered is the correct one
- Estimate the answer in your head and compare this with the answer the calculator gives. They should be approximately the same
- Check how the calculator you are going to use performs multiple options. This is particularly important when you are using a calculator in a clinical area
- Make sure that you enter the calculations in the right order. This is important when carrying out calculations involving addition/ subtraction and multiplication/division
- Make sure that the answer makes sense in the context of the calculation, e.g. when using a calculation to find the number of tablets to give to a patient. If your answer is 12 tablets, this should make you question your calculation as this a large number of tablets to take. When deciding whether to round up/down, remember that money should be rounded either up or down to the nearest penny/pound, whereas answers about numbers of people should be in whole numbers.

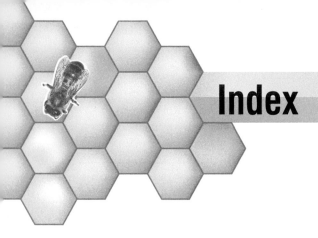

Index

A page number in **bold** type indicates a Keyword definition of the term. Page numbers in *italic* type indicate relevant numbered figures and tables.